Common Reptile Diseases and Treatment

Common Reptile Diseases and Treatment

Shawn P. Messonnier, D.V.M.

Paws & Claws Animal Hospital
Plano, Texas

**Blackwell
Science**

Blackwell Science
Editorial offices:
238 Main Street, Cambridge,
  Massachusetts 02142, USA
Osney Mead, Oxford OX2 0El,
  England
25 John Street, London WC1N 2BL,
  England
23 Ainslie Place, Edinburgh EH3 6AJ,
  Scotland
54 University Street, Carlton, Victoria
  3053, Australia

Other Editorial Offices:
Arnette Blackwell SA, 224, Boulevard
  Saint Germain, 75007 Paris, France
Blackwell Wissenschafts-Verlag
  GmbH Kurfürstendamm 57, 10707
  Berlin, Germany
Zehetnergasse 6, A-1140 Vienna,
  Austria

Distributors:
USA
  Blackwell Science, Inc.
  238 Main Street
  Cambridge, Massachusetts 02142
  (Telephone orders: 800-215-1000 or
  617-876-7000; Fax orders: 617-492-
  5263)

Canada
  Copp Clark, Ltd.
  2775 Matheson Blvd. East
  Mississauga, Ontario
  Canada, L4W 4P7
  (Telephone orders: 800-263-4374 or
  905-238-6074)

Australia
  Blackwell Science Pty., Ltd.
  54 University street
  Carlton, Victoria 3053
  (Telephone orders: 03-9347-0300;
  fax orders 03-9349 3016)

Outside North America and
Australia
  Blackwell Science, Ltd.
  c/o Marston Book Services, Ltd.
  P.O. Box 269
  Abingdon
  Oxford OX14 4YN
  England
  (Telephone orders: 44-01235-
  465500; fax orders 44-01235-465555)

Acquisitions: Jane Humphreys

Production: Ellen Samia

Typeset by Best-Set Typesetter Ltd.

Printed and bound by Walsworth
  Publishing Co.

© 1996 by Blackwell Science, Inc.

Printed in the United States of
  America

96 97 98 99 5 4 3 2 1

Library of Congress Cataloging in Publication Data
Messonnier, Shawn.
  Common reptile diseases and treatment/
  Shawn P. Messonnier. p. cm.
  Includes bibliographical references and index.
  ISBN 0-86542-553-1
  1. Captive reptiles--Diseases. 2. Pet Medicine.
    I. Title SF997.5.R4M47 1996
  639.3'9--dc20   96-32365 CIP

Contents

▼ ▼ ▼ ▼ ▼ ▼ ▼ ▼

Preface

▼　　▼　　▼　　▼　　▼　　▼　　▼　　▼

D ESPITE the popularity of reptiles as pets, it is difficult to acquire information about their medical problems and the treatment of these problems. Yes, there are some excellent reference texts that every reptile practitioner should own and use. Unfortunately, these texts are not very handy (and are, in fact, quite cumbersome) when information is needed quickly. Busy practitioners don't have time to spend precious minutes looking through several chapters for a quick answer when Mrs. Jones' snake isn't eating. Time is of the essence. Later, when time is available, the practitioner can review the pathophysiology and various etiologies of anorexia in one of the reference texts.

Common Reptile Diseases and Treatment is written with the busy practitioner in mind. The information presented covers the most common problems of the most popular reptile species kept as pets in the author's practice. As a working practitioner who sees many cases (most on a referral basis), I know what it's like to waste time trying to find a drug dose, the proper treatment, or a quick review of a procedure. This book is *the* handbook I use in my busy practice for quickly referencing vitally important information. It's not a book that should sit on your shelf collecting dust. I hope that you will use it frequently, even daily, when you need to find answers *quickly* to the most common problems you face in practice. Armed with the information in *Common Reptile Diseases and Treatment*, you can confidently treat more than 90% of the diseases you'll commonly encounter in the most popular reptile pets. For those "weird" cases, or to review useful pathophysiological or etiological information, by all means continue with your education. Attend meetings, subscribe to and read various journals and newsletters (*Exotic Pet Practice,* published monthly by Mosby, is extremely helpful), and dust off those bulky reference texts sitting on your shelves. For quick answers to routine problems, confidently reach for *Common Reptile Diseases and Treatment.*

Acknowledgments

▼   ▼   ▼   ▼   ▼   ▼   ▼   ▼

FIRST, I must thank the veterinarians who refer all of the reptile patients we see at my hospital. I always appreciate your confidence in our medical and surgical skills; I'm glad we've been able to help your clients and their sick reptile pets.

Second, I must collectively acknowledge all of the practicing doctors who treat reptile patients. Thanks for all of your advice to myself and to other exotic pet veterinarians. Through your writings and lectures, we all benefit from the exchange of knowledge.

Third, as always, a big "Thank You" and "I Love You" to my wife Sandy and daughter Erica. Writing is something I enjoy doing but it does take time. Occasionally I get irritated and moody if things don't go "just right." Thanks for your constant love and support. My writing is as much for you as it is for me; thank you for just being you.

Finally, to the great folks at Blackwell, especially Maya Crosby, who saw the importance of this project and helped get it off the ground, and Jane Humphreys, who continued working with me on the project. I'm looking forward to working with you folks again in the future.

Shawn P. Messonnier, D.V.M.

Introduction to Reptile Medicine

▼   ▼   ▼   ▼   ▼   ▼   ▼   ▼

R EPTILES are popular pets. Some people want to own them to be different (never a good sole reason for owning any pet), some people enjoy the lower cost of veterinary care associated with owning a reptile than with owning a dog or cat (a perception that is often, but not totally, true), and many people who don't have the time to devote to a dog or cat enjoy the relatively "maintenance-free" appeal of a snake, iguana, or turtle.

Prior to owning a reptile, every prospective owner would do well to meet with a knowledgeable veterinarian to discuss his or her interest. Many owners who purchase reptiles probably have no business owning such a pet. Unfortunately, these prepurchase consultations rarely occur. If you are fortunate enough to meet with a client who is considering owning a reptile, I would advise you to pose the following questions to him or her:

1. Do you want a pet just to look at it, or do you want to handle and socialize with it?

While many reptiles, especially those purchased as captive-born infants, allow owners to handle them, others do not. Many of the more exotic species such as chameleons do not allow handling and react aggressively or become severely stressed. As a rule, if you want to snuggle with your pet, a reptile is not for you. If, on the other hand, you want an animal you can display, a reptile would be a good consideration.

2. How much time can you devote to your pet?

This author believes that all pets require at least daily observation for a minimum of 15 minutes. The owner who fails to pay at least this much attention to his or her pet won't detect early signs of disease, and is really neglecting his or her responsibility as a pet owner. Most reptiles need to be fed and watered daily, and often the cage needs to be cleaned daily as well. The owner who intends to put a reptile in a cage and observe it only infrequently should seriously consider his or her decision to care for this type of pet.

3. Can you afford proper medical care?

All reptiles need to be examined immediately after purchase (within 48 hours) and at least annually to allow for early detection of disease. With very rare exceptions, exotic pets don't usually act sick or show any indication of illness until they are *very sick!* My staff is trained to gently tell pet owners who call to inquire about how to care for a sick reptile that any sick exotic pet isn't just sick: it's dying! Regular veterinary care, coupled with informed pet ownership, greatly reduces illness and death in these pets.

4. Can you make or buy the correct habitat (home) for your reptile?

At a minimum, reptiles require a 10-gallon glass aquarium, two pieces of astroturf to line the bottom, a source of heat, and a source of UV light (see chapter 3, "Housing"). While not expensive or difficult to assemble, improper environment is the second most common cause of diseases and captivity problems encountered in reptiles (improper diet is the most common source of problems).

Reptiles do get sick, and preventing illness is definitely preferred to treatment. At a minimum, owners need to understand that reptiles hide signs of illness quite well. This characteristic is a preservation response. In the wild, if an animal showed signs of illness whenever it felt bad, it would readily be attacked by predators or members of its own group. Therefore, these animals don't appear ill until the course of the disease is actually quite advanced. Our pet reptiles still retain this "wild" characteristic. *A sick reptile is a dying reptile!* It's very important to inform clients that their sick reptiles need to be seen by a veterinarian at the first signs of illness. Waiting to see if things get better, or treatment with over-the-counter medications, especially those sold at pet stores, only delays the proper treatment and often results in expensive veterinary bills and a dead reptile. We can do many things for sick reptiles—and not all sick reptiles are dead reptiles—but we need to start treatment early.

The reptile veterinarian needs to remember an important principle of medical practice: *treat the pet, not just the disease.* While it might be tempting to contain costs by treating a sick iguana just for metabolic bone disease, you do the pet and owner a disservice by failing to diagnose and treat the oxyurid infection that is also present. Sick reptiles often have multiple problems; a thorough diagnostic evaluation is needed in every case to identify these problems properly and to offer the owner the proper treatment regimen. While some owners may decline further diagnostic testing and consent to treating only the immediate problem, they should be offered a complete workup nevertheless.

Finally, remember that this book is not meant to be a surgical text. Throughout the discussions, some of the treatment options mentioned include surgery; consultation with additional references (Boyer, Frye, Bennett, and so forth) is needed to understand surgical approaches. Hands-on practice obtained through wet labs will greatly increase a practitioner's skill and confidence in treating surgical conditions. Until that time, referral to a more qualified reptile veterinarian is highly recommended.

Starting a Reptile Practice

▼   ▼   ▼   ▼   ▼   ▼   ▼   ▼

1

T REATING reptiles offers exciting challenges to the practitioner. Currently, very few veterinarians have the interest or qualifications to treat these exotic pets. Yet reptiles are popular pets (approximately 7 million "exotic" pets are found in the United States) and require regular veterinary care.

From a medical viewpoint, treating reptiles presents a nice diversion and challenge from the usual "dog and cat cases." These interesting pets help to break up an otherwise routine day of vaccinations, neuters, and spays. Financially, they can add to the practice and, in some cases, make up a large part of the practice. For some veterinarians, their entire practice consists of treating exotic pets (reptiles, pocket pets, and birds). Because so few veterinarians treat these pets, there is very little competition. In addition, most reptile owners will spend a significant amount of money to treat these pets. While not all owners have bottomless pockets, I've found that, compared with dog and cat owners, fewer reptile owners refuse treatment solely because of cost (although they may decline extensive workups). This attitude is refreshing, because if you enjoy diagnostic medicine, you'll enjoy working with reptiles. Most sick reptiles have as their only presenting signs anorexia and lethargy, so often a complete diagnostic workup is needed.

Many reptile owners have been shunned, treated rudely, and even laughed at by other veterinarians for wanting to spend money to treat their pets. Reptiles require the same diligent care that dogs and cats need. The fact that a pet turtle costs only $20 is immaterial to an owner who wants someone to save a dying pet. Be as proficient as possible, and always offer the best care. Let the owner decide what he or she can afford to spend on the pet's care. It is the owner's decision, not yours!

Before you even attempt to treat reptiles, you should question your motivation for undertaking this venture. Some veterinarians may have formed the impression from the last few paragraphs that I'm suggesting everyone start treating reptiles so we can all make "big bucks." That is the *worst* reason for starting a reptile practice! First, financial gain is never guaranteed with any profession or interest. Second, if you're motivated solely by money, sooner or later you'll grow tired and look for something else to do. The desire to make more money is the wrong motive, and if it represents the only reason for your interest in reptile medicine, your practice is doomed to failure.

You should have a sincere interest in wanting to treat reptiles. If you have this interest, then yes, it can be financially rewarding as well (and it should be, just like any other part of your practice).

As I've said, treating reptiles can be fun and exciting, as well as challenging. Reptile medicine is still in its infancy. The Association for Reptile and Amphibian Veterinarians (ARAV) was formed only recently. This "newness" can be both exciting and frustrating. There are some "experts" that you can contact, but very often you're on your own. As a result, it's extremely important to learn as much as possible.

Several sources of information need to be mentioned. Dr. Frederic Frye has written what many consider the "bible" for reptile veterinarians. His book, *Biomedical and Surgical Aspects of Captive Reptile Husbandry*, should be found on the shelf of every serious reptile practitioner. Consider contacting a local veterinary school to see if any recent class lecture notes are available for purchase. Dr. Murray Fowler's book *Zoo and Wild Animal Medicine* is a useful reference as well. I would strongly recommend joining the ARAV to keep up with current developments in the field. In addition, Mosby publishes a monthly publication on the care and treatment of exotic pets called *Exotic Pet Practice* that is specifically geared for the practitioner. Finally, consider becoming a member of the Chicago Herpetological Society, as well as any local herp societies.

■ **EQUIPMENT/SUPPLIES/PHARMACEUTICALS**

You won't need much new equipment to begin treating reptiles, especially if you already treat birds. I list some of the essentials for treating reptiles in the following sections.

Antibiotics

Many bacterial infections in reptiles are caused by gram-negative organisms. Enrofloxacin, amikacin, piperacillin, and trimethoprim-sulfa are commonly employed for these infections. Metronidazole is often used, both for its appetite-stimulating properties (in anorectic snakes) and for its efficacy against protozoal and anaerobic infections (as many as 50% of infections in reptiles are caused by anaerobic organisms). Enrofloxacin should be reserved for severe, life-threatening cases or resistant infections. Usually, antibiotics are given in injectable, rather than oral, forms because of the difficulty of administering oral medications to reptiles. Absorption of oral antibiotics can be erratic and unpredictable in sick reptiles. In addition, severe gram-negative infections usually require an aminoglycoside, which is available only in an injectable form. Most owners can easily be taught to medicate their pets with injectable medications.

Miscellaneous Medications

Metronidazole, ivermectin, and fenbendazole are commonly used anthelmintics. Injacom-100 or Injacom-100 B is often used in the supportive care of sick reptiles, but especially in iguanas suffering from metabolic bone disease because of the vitamin D content of the medication. Many practitioners use ascorbic acid (vitamin C) when treating infectious stomatitis. Oxytocin and various forms of calcium are used for the rare instances of dystocia (arginine vasopressin is reportedly effective but is currently unavailable; in addition, its use is controversial). Calcium is commonly used to treat metabolic bone disease, with calcitonin being used to treat this condition in iguanas. Isoflurane is a safe inhalant anesthetic (and the only anesthetic I use routinely in my reptile practice), although ketamine works well for sedation in some species. Emeraid II (Lafeber) is my choice for force-feeding supplementation, although other foods can be mixed with this (see chapter 5, "Clinical Procedures").

Needles and Syringes

Because of the dilutions used when treating reptiles, 1/2 mL TB syringes with 27- or 28-gauge needles are convenient (Fig. 1.1).

Feeding Tubes

Various sizes of red rubber tubes work well, both for force feeding and for cloacal washes or enemas (see Fig. 1.2). For small reptiles (<100 g), plastic tom cat urinary catheters work well for these procedures.

Doppler Devices

Doppler devices are used instead of stethoscopy in reptiles. Doppler devices have greater sensitivity, are often easier to use, and avoid the interference from skin and scales that often presents a problem with stethoscopy (1). Two units are especially effective: the Ultrascope Obstetrical Doppler, Model 2, 2.25 MHz, and the Ultrascope Doppler

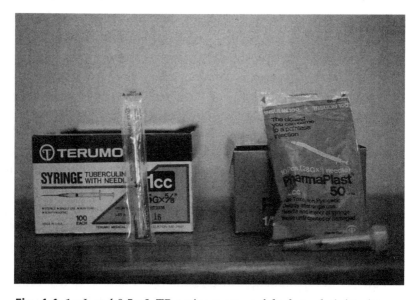

Fig. 1.1 *1 mL and 0.5 mL TB syringes are useful when administering medications to reptiles.*

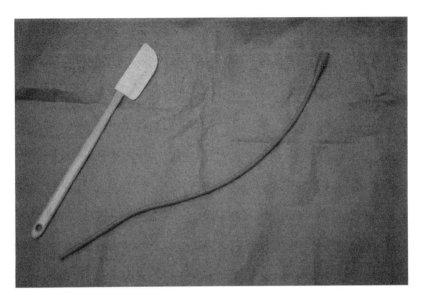

Fig. 1.2 *A red rubber tube and rubber spatula are used for force-feeding reptiles.*

Arterial and Venous Blood Flow Detector, Model 8, 8 MHz. Both are available from EMS Products, Inc., Kirkland, Washington.

Sexing Probes

Metallic probes of various sizes can be used when sexing snakes and iguanas. Alternatively, tom cat catheters and red rubber feeding tubes can be used. Lubricants such as K-Y jelly should be used to make the procedure more comfortable for the reptile.

Plastic Spatulas

Plastic spatulas are handy for *gently* opening the mouth of a snake or iguana. Paper clips, when used gently, work well for small turtles. I occasionally have some difficulty in opening a turtle's mouth. As a threat display (or a defensive posture), the turtle may open its mouth voluntarily if you place your hand near its head, allowing a quick inspection.

Incubators

Most sick reptiles are hypothermic. A used human pediatric incubator (see Fig. 1.3) works well when hospitalization is required; several companies make heated aquaria for the same purpose. I routinely maintain sick reptiles at 85–95 °F depending upon the species of pet (85–90 °F for snakes and turtles, 90–100 °F for iguanas). Owners who refuse hospitalization and opt for home treatment should keep their reptiles at this same temperature; correct environmental temperature is critical in treating serious reptile illnesses to allow maximal functioning of the immune system.

Gram Scales

Gram scales are useful when weighing smaller reptiles. Battery or electronic scales also work well. Because weight gain or loss may be the first or only sign of illness, reptiles should be weighed at every visit.

Surgical Instruments

Small size is important for surgical instruments, as reptile patients are usually smaller than most dogs and cats. Iris scissors, small hemostats, tissue forceps, jeweler's forceps, small scissors, and nee-

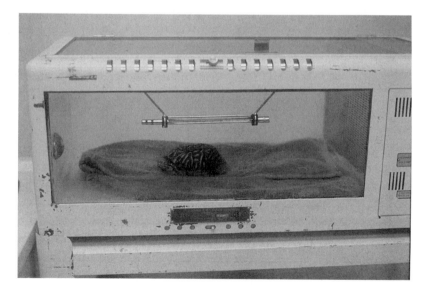

Fig. 1.3 *Used human pediatric incubators can often be purchased inexpensively and are ideal for providing the warmth required by sick reptiles.*

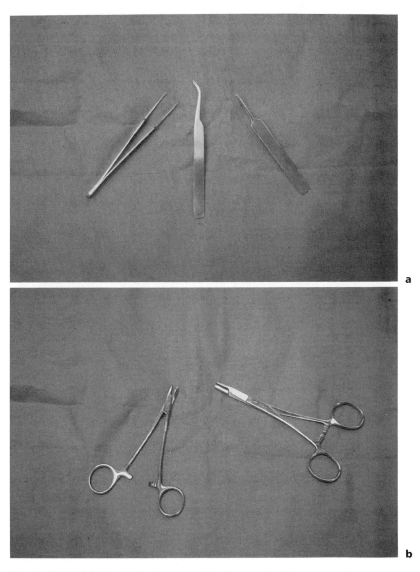

Fig. 1.4(a & b) *Jeweler's forceps and microsurgical instruments are handy for reptile surgery.*

dle holders make your job much easier (see Fig. 1.4), as does a good light source. Fine suture material, such as 3-0–6-0 Vicryl or PDS works well. Vicryl, Dexon, and PDS are preferred over chromic gut because of the intense inflammatory response seen with gut. Nylon

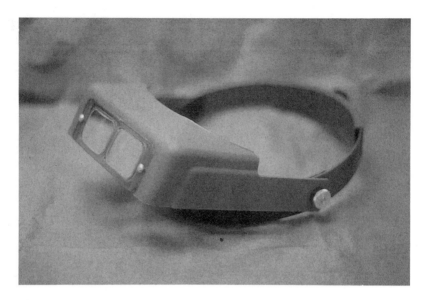

Fig. 1.5 *Extra magnification is inexpensively provided by an OptiVisor.*

or polypropylene is preferred when suturing skin (2). An everting pattern is preferred to prevent inversion of the skin (2).

Because skin heals slowly in reptiles, sutures are usually not removed until 4–6 weeks postoperatively, or until the next shed occurs at the surgical site (2, 3). Healing time is decreased if incisions are made between—rather than through—scales (2).

Depending upon your eyesight, magnification with an operating microscope or OptiVisor (see Fig. 1.5) may be needed.

■ REFERENCES

1. Frye F. Ultrasonic Doppler blood flow detection in small exotic animal medicine. Seminars in avian and exotic pet medicine, July 1990; 3:133–139.
2. Faulkner J, Archambault A. Anesthesia and surgery in green iguanas. Seminars in avian and exotic pet medicine, April 1993; 2:103–108.
3. Bennett RA. Reptilian surgery part I. Basic principles. Compend Contin Educ Pract Vet, January 1989; 11:10–18.

Marketing

▼   ▼   ▼   ▼   ▼   ▼   ▼   ▼

I F YOU have the strong, sincere interest and desire to treat reptiles, you obviously need to make this fact known to potential clients. Every business does marketing. Even though this word has left a bad taste in many doctors' mouths because of its unfortunate association with "low cost" shot clinics and "Free Exam" coupons, marketing is necessary if you want to treat reptiles. Most of your practice will take place on a referral basis, although occasionally a client may call inquiring to see if you treat reptiles. To generate referrals, you need to let potential sources of referrals know about your special skills and interests.

Referrals come from several sources. Local veterinarians are a major source that must be cultivated. Let area doctors know about your special interest in this field. All veterinarians receive calls from clients looking for someone to treat their sick reptiles. Make sure other doctors refer these clients to you!

When I began treating exotic pets, I had cultivated good relationships with other veterinarians in the area. If you've never met the colleague down the street, you really can't expect him or her to refer people to you. You may have already made some friendships with local veterinarians. I sent each veterinarian in the area a letter describing my background education and experience with reptiles. I asked them to refer any clients to me that called with a sick reptile. An important part of my letter pointed out that I was *not* interested in "stealing" or seeing these clients for any reason other than treatment of their sick reptiles. Many owners of exotic pets also own a dog or cat, and I wanted my fellow colleagues to know that I would refer these people back to them for their continued care of the dog and cat patients. In fact, I haven't even had any clients ask questions about their other pets. In summary, you need to obtain referrals from your colleagues, and a letter asking for referrals is a great way to start.

I also contacted a local veterinary association and put my name on a list of doctors with experience in treating exotics; I have since received a few referrals from them. Our local zoo maintains a list of veterinarians with experience in dealing with exotic pets, so I was placed on their list as well. It's interesting that many people with an exotic pet call the zoo asking for a veterinary referral.

Because you may already treat reptiles, you probably know that pet stores receive many inquiries about the care and treatment of reptiles. I'm always amazed that pet stores often seem to be the first source from which a pet owner seeks answers to pet care questions, when in reality so many of these stores have not adequately trained their employees. Often the advice given by the employees is not only incorrect, but also dangerous! I strongly urge you to make contact with area pet stores, even those that don't sell reptiles, as they often field calls from owners. Let the area stores know that they can call you for free advice whenever they need it. I also encourage store personnel to have an owner call right from the store if possible with any questions. To educate store employees, consider giving pet stores handouts on the care of reptiles. In Addition, an in-store "seminar" is very helpful.

In addition, local herp clubs can be a good source of clients. Speaking at their meetings, writing for their newsletters, or advertising in the newsletters will put your name in front of the public.

As you can see, there are several groups you need to contact for referrals. Without marketing, it's almost impossible to build any kind of reptile practice. Once you become known, however, you'll see reptiles on a regular basis. To keep the referrals coming, consider sending a newsletter to your referral sources. The newsletter can highlight a few of the more interesting cases you have seen as a result of the referrals. My newsletter, the *Avian/Exotic Newsletter*, is mailed twice a year to approximately 100 area veterinarians, clubs, pet stores, and groomers. This activity is the only marketing I undertake for the exotic side of my practice, and it is extremely effective and inexpensive. Letting others know the type of care available for sick reptiles will increase their confidence in you and encourage continued referrals.

Housing

▼　　▼　　▼　　▼　　▼　　▼　　▼　　▼

3

S MALL reptiles often do well in 10- to 20-gallon aquariums, whereas larger animals must be moved to more comfortable enclosures. These cages can often be purchased or built by the pet owner. At a minimum, the pet should be able to turn around in the cage; snakes should be able to stretch to at least one-quarter to one-half of the body length.

Substrate (cage lining material) should be easy to clean and non-toxic to reptiles. Newspaper, butcher's paper, cloth towels, paper towels, or astroturf is recommended (1–5). Astroturf is preferred by many reptile owners. The owner should acquire two pieces and cut them to fit the bottom of the cage. One piece is placed in the cage, while the other piece is kept outside and thus is always clean. When the turf inside the cage becomes soiled, the owner will then have a clean, dry piece to replace it. The soiled turf can be cleaned with ordinary soap and water (dilute bleach, dilute chlorhexidine solution, or dilute Roccal can also be used as long as the cage and turf are properly rinsed), thoroughly rinsed, and hung to dry before the next cage cleaning.

Alfalfa pellets can also be used as bedding for iguanas or turtles; these pellets are often eaten by the pet without problems. Owners should avoid sand, gravel, wood shavings, corn cob material, walnut shells, mud, moss, and cat litter, as these substances are harder to clean and can cause impactions if eaten on purpose or accidentally if the food becomes covered by these substrates (1–5). In particular, cedar wood shavings are reportedly toxic to reptiles.

Natural branches are enjoyed by both snakes and iguanas. Owners must ensure that they are secure and won't fall onto the pet and cause an injury. Ideally, the branch should slope from the bottom of the enclosure to the top, ending near a heat source so that the pet can bask. Large rocks in the cage also allow for basking. A hiding place is appreciated by all reptiles; reptiles without hiding boxes often become stressed and ill. Artificial plants can be arranged to provide hiding spaces, as can clay pots, cardboard boxes, and other containers that provide a secure area. In general, reptiles should receive 12 hours of light and 12 hours of darkness each day (5).

■ HEATING

A heat source is necessary for all reptiles, as reptiles are ectothermic and need a variety of temperatures to regulate their internal temperature. Ideally, the cage should be set up so that a heat gradient is established, with one area of the tank being warmer than the other end. In this way, the pet can move around its environment and warm or cool itself as needed. To establish and maintain the proper temperature gradient, owners should purchase two thermometers and place one at the cooler end and one at the warmer end. The cooler end of the cage should be approximately 70–75 °F, while the warmer end should be 90–95 °F for most reptiles (1–5). As a guideline, approximate temperature ranges are: iguanas, 75–100 °F; ball pythons, 75–90 °F; and box turtles, 70–90 °F (1–5). Several veterinarians and herpetologists feel that box turtles can remain healthy if nighttime temperatures in the spring, summer, and fall approach the low 50s; obviously, daytime warming is needed to prevent pseudohibernation (see chapter 8, "Diseases and Treatment of Turtles"). Temperatures may vary for exotic species, and a reference book should be consulted for information.

A convenient, inexpensive, and safe way to supply heat is with a focal heat source. A 100 W incandescent bulb with a reflector hood works well. This heat source should be placed *outside* and above one end of the cage, which should be covered by a screen top to prevent iguanas and snakes from escaping or burning themselves on the bulb. At night, additional heat usually isn't necessary as long as the temperature remains 65–70 °F. If additional heat is needed, room space heaters, heating pads placed under an elevated cage (elevated about 1 in. off the surface), or infrared bulbs can be used. In place of or in addition to 100 W light bulbs, ceramic heating bulbs can be used (contact Repticare Light, ZooMed, 3090 McMillan Rd., San Luis Obispo, California 93401, or Pearlco Lights, Habitat Creations, 516-736-9587).

A good way to allow the reptile to bask is to place the bulb and hood at one end of the cage and arrange a branch or perching (basking) area near the light. This set-up allows the animal psychological stimulation (provided by the climbing) as well as a safe heat source.

A popular form of offering heat for reptiles is the infamous "Hot Rock" or "Sizzle Rock." These devices are dangerous and should be avoided! With the exception of very small reptiles, they will not adequately supply enough heat for the pet. Even if the owner can find a large enough rock, it is hard to locate one that is safe. Many stories are told of reptiles burning themselves, often severely, from prolonged contact with this heat source (and others). Why an animal would not remove itself from a dangerously hot object is unknown, but it is not uncommon for reptiles to sustain severe, even fatal, burns from a Hot Rock. Therefore, these external sources of heat are not recommended.

As mentioned earlier, heating pads can be used underneath the cage, at one end of the enclosure. Owners should be advised to make sure that the pad adequately warms that part of the cage and to ensure that it doesn't overheat the cage, creating a "greenhouse effect." Many experts recommend elevating the cage about 1 in. off the ground with blocks and then sliding the heating pad underneath the cage. If heating pads are used, the top of the cage must not be open or too much heat will be lost (5). A few small holes can be cut at the top and along the lower part of the cage for ventilation and some thermoregulation.

Heating tape or coils of the variety used to warm the soil for plant protection present another possibility. Such heat sources need to be buried in soil (soil usually isn't recommended as a cage substrate) and can cause harm if exposed (5).

Finally, space room heaters can be used if the room cools down too much at night. They probably shouldn't be the only heat source, as they don't allow for a cooler area of the cage.

■ UV LIGHT

A source of vitamin D₃ must also be provided. Lack of vitamin D_3 is a major cause of metabolic bone disease. While vitamin D_3 certainly should be provided in the diet, it is still necessary to provide it to reptiles by using UV light, especially since some question remains as to whether some reptiles (iguanas) can absorb dietary vitamin D_3. In addition to providing vitamin D_3, these lights, as well as full-spectrum lights, seem to have a positive impact on the psychological well-being of the pet.

The best recommendation is to provide the UV light using a two-bulb fixture. The lights should be within 6–12 in. of the pet for maximum effectiveness. Ideally, the UV light should emit light in the UV-B range (290–320 nm) (5, 6). Combining a blacklight (such as the blacklight blue from General Electric) with a Vita-Lite, Chroma-50, or Colortone-50 in a two-bulb fixture seems to meet the needs of the pet. Other acceptable UV lights include TL-09 and TL-12 from Philips, and the Ultra-Vitalux from Osram.* The plant blacklight from Sylvania, the Gro-lux, definitely needs to be combined with a UV light. Because the output of UV lights decreases with age, many experts recommend replacing the lights every 6–12 months. For UV lights to supply adequate vitamin D_3, the light must reach the pet unfiltered, so no glass or plastic should be interposed between the pet and the light (a screen or mesh covering on the top of the cage allows the UV light to enter and prevents the reptiles from escaping). Some manufacturers sell cages constructed of material that supposedly does not filter UV light. According to their package inserts, however, UV light in the critical 290–320 nm range is filtered, making these cages useless for reptiles.

Plant lights (without additional UV light supplementation) and poster blacklights are not recommended, as they don't provide much light in the 290–320 nm range.

Exposing the pet to direct, unfiltered sunlight is always a good idea. Several words of caution should be given, however. First, the

*Other companies that manufacture UV-B lights include Energy Savers (310-784-2770), Luminram (914-698-1205), and ZooMed (San Luis Obispo, California). Owners should check and make sure that the lights they purchase provide UV light in the correct spectrum as mentioned in the text.

UV light of sunlight is filtered by plastic or glass. Second, putting a glass aquarium in direct sunlight can easily cause the habitat to become dangerously hot (similar to leaving a child or pet in a closed car in the summer). Third, taking the pet out of its normal cage is fine, but care must be given to prevent its escape or attack by other pets. An outdoor cage constructed of wood and wire screen is an acceptable method of exposing reptiles to sunlight. Fourth, some reptiles become aggressive immediately following exposure to sunlight.

■ OUTDOOR HOUSING (TURTLES)

Some owners may inquire about outdoor housing for their pet turtles. Many turtles do well outdoors in the warmer months. For their own protection, they should be contained within an enclosure. A shaded area, as well as a hiding area, should be provided. Turtles can dig out of enclosures, so fencing should be buried 6–12 in. or bricks or rocks placed under the area. Some owners find a child's wading pool a suitable environment. Astroturf can be used for lining material, or grass, twigs, and other natural materials will be fine *if* they are changed daily. Of course, food and water must be available. The turtle should be brought indoors when temperature drops below 60 °F. Finally, owners should be warned that turtles can become prey for dogs and cats; they should exercise care when housing a turtle outdoors.

■ HIBERNATING (7)

As a rule, non-breeding snakes and iguanas don't usually need to hibernate if the ambient temperature remains in their comfort zone. On the other hand, many turtles will hibernate if given the opportunity. Hibernating is a controversial topic among reptile veterinarians. I usually advise against it, unless the pet has had a thorough physical examination, appropriate laboratory tests are conducted prior to hibernation to ensure health, and the owner constructs the hibernaculum and will monitor the turtle during hibernation. Many veterinarians do not consider hibernation essential for a turtle's well-being, but some owners wish to provide conditions for hibernation. Hibernation is felt to be essential for adequate reproduction if the turtle will be used for breeding. If the ambient temperature remains warm, some turtles may stop eating in the fall; many will continue feeding and skip hibernation, however.

As noted, only turtles that are in good health should be allowed to hibernate, so a thorough examination and laboratory tests are essential prior to hibernation (an examination and microscopic fecal examination should be performed at minimum). Turtles must also be allowed free access to food prior to hibernation.

If an owner elects hibernation, it usually begins in the fall (September or October). As the temperature drops, especially if the cage temperature is allowed to cool, the turtle may decrease its feeding. At this time, food—but not water—should be withheld for 1–2 weeks and the temperature kept at 70–80 °F. The turtle can then eliminate and clear its gastrointestinal tract. After this period, remove the external heat source for a week and allow the turtle to remain at room temperature (60–70 °F). The turtle can then be placed in its hibernating compartment (hibernaculum).

The hibernaculum should have dim light and the temperature should remain at 50–60 °F. An occasional drop to 45 °F is acceptable. *Persistent temperatures above 60 °F are not cool enough for hibernation and allow the turtle to turn up its metabolism and slowly starve (see chapter 8).* Temperatures below 45 °F are detrimental as well. For the safety of the turtle, it should not be allowed to hibernate outdoors where environmental temperature and predators can't be monitored.

The hibernaculum should have a foot of humid peat-based potting soil and a 3–6 in. layer of shredded newspaper, leaves, or hay on top, allowing the turtle to burrow. The soil should remain damp, but not wet, to prevent the turtle from dehydrating. A small water bowl should be present to prevent dehydration. As a rule, turtles will hibernate for 3–5 months. Any turtle that appears ill during hibernation should be examined. The owner should check the turtle weekly at minimum. Pneumonia may be detected; signs of this disease include nasal discharge, mucus in the oral cavity, and gurgling respiratory sounds.

At the end of the hibernating period, the turtle should be placed into its regular cage and the temperature slowly warmed to the normal range over a 1-week period. Food should then be offered.

■ **REFERENCES**

1. Messonnier SP. Exotic pets: A veterinary guide for owners. Plano, Texas: Wordware 1995.

2. De Vosjoli P. The general care and maintenance of the green iguana. Lakeside: Advanced Vivarium Series, 1990:9–18.

3. De Vosjoli P. The general care and maintenance of ball pythons. Lakeside: Advanced Vivarium Series, 1990:11–14.

4. De Vosjoli P. The general care and maintenance of box turtles. Lakeside: Advanced Vivarium Series, 1991:10–14.

5. Frye F. Reptile care: An atlas of diseases and treatments, vols. I and II. Neptune City, NJ: TFH, 1991.

6. Boyer T. Common problems and treatments of green iguanas (*Iguana iguana*). Bull of ARAV, Premiere Issue, 1991:8–11.

7. Boyer T. Box turtle care. Bull of ARAV, Premiere Issue, 1991:14–16.

Feeding

▼   ▼   ▼   ▼   ▼   ▼   ▼   ▼

4

■ IGUANAS

In feeding green iguanas (1), it is important to understand how these reptiles feed in the wild. The green iguana is a reptile native to Central and South America and Mexico. Studies in Panama found that the iguana eats mainly vegetable matter, including the fruit, leaves, and flowers of certain bushes, trees, and vines, with feeding occurring in frequent, small meals. Thus, iguanas are mainly herbivorous, although they may eat insects in small amounts. Their diet mainly consists of fiber and plant protein, and contains very little fat. The iguana's hindgut is highly specialized to allow fiber digestion, similar to the stomach compartments of cattle.

Currently, two schools of thought exist about the proper feeding regimen of iguanas. Some doctors and herpetologists recommend a diet consisting of 100% plant-based matter. Others recommend a diet consisting of 80–90% plant-based matter with 10–20% animal-based protein, such as crickets, worms, and moths (if the iguana will eat these insects). Until the controversy can be solved, the individual practitioner will need to make his or her own recommendations. Regardless of which recommendation is offered to the client, the importance of a mainly vegetable diet should be stressed.

For veterinarians recommending animal-based protein with a mainly plant-based diet, the following regimens are recommended. Two different feeding regimens for iguanas are offered, one for juveniles (younger than 2 years of age) and one for adults (older than 2 years of age), as the nutritional requirements are presumed to be slightly different in growing animals versus adults. For juvenile iguanas, 80% of their diet should be plant-based protein material

23
▼

and 20% animal-based protein material. For adult iguanas, 90% of the diet should be plant-based and 10% animal-based. This decrease in animal protein will help prevent gout and renal failure. Of the plant matter, most (80%) should be vegetable- or flower-based, and only 20% fruit-based. Even though iguanas enjoy the sweetness of fruit, it is mineral-deficient compared with vegetables. Fruit should mainly be considered a treat.

Plant-based matter acceptable for iguanas includes the following items. As a rule, anything green and leafy should make up a large part of the diet. Yellow and orange vegetables should also be included. Fiber-rich, vitamin- and mineral-deficient vegetables such as lettuce and celery should be avoided (small amounts of romaine lettuce can be offered as part of the vegetable "salad"). Owners should be told that a pet eating lettuce and celery is no different from the owners eating paper or cardboard, as the composition of these two vegetables is mainly fiber and water with little vitamins or minerals.

Acceptable vegetables include collard/mustard/turnip greens, alfalfa chow or hay, bok choy, kale, parsley, spinach (less than 10% of the vegetable matter, as spinach contains oxalates that bind calcium), bell pepper, green beans, green peas, corn, okra, cactus, yellow squash/zucchini/acorn squash, sweet potatoes, cabbage, broccoli, and flowers such as carnations, hibiscus, and roses (azaleas are toxic and should be avoided). Table 4.1 lists the calcium content of some vegetables commonly used as reptile food. Flowers, their stems, and leaves can be offered to the iguana. Because I have treated several iguanas with impactions caused by eating a large amount of stems, I recommend limiting this part of the plant. Vegetables can be offered either cooked or raw. The owner should experiment with the iguana to see if it prefers raw or cooked food. Flowers can be home-grown or purchased from floral shops. Floral shops often throw out older, wilting flowers that may be unacceptable for sale to the public, but which reptile owners can sometimes obtain for free. It is prudent to ensure that no chemicals have been recently applied to the flowers or their water containers, however. Flowers, vegetables, and fruits should be thoroughly washed prior to feeding.

Fruit can include apples, pears, bananas, grapes, peaches, kiwi, and melons. Especially good are figs (which contain more calcium than other fruits), papayas, raspberries, and strawberries.

Appropriate animal-based protein sources include crickets, sardines (drained), tofu, hard-boiled eggs, earthworms, and mealworms. Dog food and cat food contain too much vitamin D and fat, and should never be fed to iguanas. (Some veterinarians feel that dog food is acceptable if it accounts for less than 5% of the iguana's diet.

Table 4.1 *Calcium Content of Common Reptile Foods (100 g sample)*

Apple	6.0 mg
Green beans	56 mg
Broccoli	88 mg
Carrot tops	310 mg
Alfalfa (dry)	1700 mg
Potato	5 mg
Iceburg lettuce	19 mg
Celery	20 mg
Squash (many varieties)	28 mg
Sweet potato	29 mg
Lima beans	52 mg
Romaine lettuce	67 mg
Spinach	93 mg
Fescue grass	130 mg
Dandelion greens	187 mg
Collard greens	203 mg
Parsley	203 mg
Turnip greens	246 mg
Kale	249 mg
Opuntia cactus	1890 mg

Adapted from Atlas of Nutritional Data of United States and Canadian Feeds, National Academy of Science, Washington, D.C., 1971, and Adams, C.F., Agricultural handbook #456, Nutritive Value of American Foods in Common Units, 1975.

While I do not disagree, I don't trust owners to limit the dog food to 5% or less and, therefore, tell owners not to use this food at all.) Reptile pellets, bird pellets, trout chow, and other fish chows are an excellent animal-based protein source; providing these substances precludes the need for live prey (although you can feed live prey, such as crickets, as the iguana may enjoy the psychological stimulation of catching the live prey).

Live prey, such as crickets and worms, should be either raised by the owner or purchased from a pet store or reptile breeder. *Never* feed an iguana insects taken from the family garden. Raising insects is easy; the Chicago Herpetological Society published an excellent manual entitled *The Right Way to Feed Insect-Eating Lizards* that discusses this topic. If owners get their insects from a local pet store, it is a good idea to "nutrient load" them prior to feeding the insects to the iguana. Keep these insects in a container and feed them finely ground rodent or fish chow or fish flakes blended with calcium carbonate powder (if using fish flakes, add high-protein baby cereal flakes). A slice of orange (for crickets) or sweet potato (mealworms) can serve as a water source for the insects. Insects should be fed for at least a few days prior to offering them to the iguana. Before feeding the iguana, the owner should lightly sprinkle the insects with a good multivitamin powder. One ground multivitamin tablet (such as Centrum) lightly sprinkled on the food each day is also acceptable.

To ensure the proper amounts of vitamins and minerals in the diet, the owner should *lightly* sprinkle all food offered to the iguana with a calcium powder (such as ground calcium gluconate, lactate, or carbonate tablets). Weekly, a *light* sprinkling of a good reptile vitamain on the food is also recommended. A *light* dusting means just that—oversupplementation can cause problems. Hypervitaminosis D is a common occurrence in pets oversupplemented with vitamins. It can be avoided by holding back on the supplementation. Remember that supplementation is truly necessary only if the animal is not eating a well-balanced diet. Well-balanced diets probably do not require supplementation. Because most owners do not feed well-balanced diets, light supplementation may be a necessity. Owners should think of a light sprinkling the same way they would *lightly* salt food for themselves.

Juvenile iguanas should be fed daily, while adult iguanas can be fed every other day. These recommendations are just guidelines, however, and many adult iguanas will eat daily.

Fresh water, offered in a crock that won't easily tip over, should be available at all times. Iguanas not only will drink from the water bowl but will often bathe in it as well (although it is perfectly acceptable to mist the iguana a few times a week). Owners must make sure the water stays clean (many reptiles love to eliminate in their water dish).

In summary, iguanas eat mainly plant-based food. Variety is the key. Owners should not let their iguanas get "hooked" on just one or two favorite items; they should feed many items in small portions. The food pieces should be cut into the proper size for the pet: smaller iguanas need their food finely chopped. As with all pets, fresh vegetables are preferred, frozen is second best, and canned is least desirable. Owners can make up about a week's worth of the diet and refrigerate or freeze the rest for convenience. A pet is what it eats and, when feeding on insects, the pet is what its prey eats; prey should be fed properly, too!

■ BALL PYTHONS

Snakes eat live or killed prey. While this regimen simplifies things for snake owners, and almost totally prevents the dietary-related diseases so commonly seen in other reptiles, it does present a problem. Namely, prey must be provided for the snake. If a client is squeamish about killing rodents for the snake and watching it eat, then a snake probably is not the best choice of pet!

Ideally, the snake should be provided with a thawed, previously frozen prey or a freshly killed prey item. It is not recommended to feed live prey to the snake for several reasons. First, the prey obviously knows it's prey; unless killed and eaten immediately, it certainly suffers some psychological stress. Second, and surprising for many snake owners, is the fact that even a small mouse can severely injure and kill a snake if the snake isn't hungry! For humane reasons, it's best to supply dead prey. The only exception would occur when the owner knows that the snake will immediately kill and eat the prey, and the owner is *constantly* observing the snake and prey until the prey is eaten or removed from the cage. Even so, a slight possibility exists of injury to the snake. Unweaned (infant) prey are safe to feed alive.

The most common prey are mice or rats. Many ball pythons won't eat these animals, however, as their diet in the wild consists of gerbils and various African species of rats and not these other rodents so commonly available in pet stores. Ball pythons often refuse to feed for months. Getting one to start eating takes patience and often the assistance of a reptile veterinarian.

A healthy ball python can go for months without eating without ill effects. Before deciding that the anorexia is normal, a physical exam and appropriate lab tests (at least a stool check for internal parasites) are recommended.

To help clients to induce their snakes to eat, the following general protocol is advised for working with the anorectic snake:

1. Discuss the environment during the first veterinary visit. If a proper heat source or hiding place is lacking, these problems need to be corrected.
2. Examine the snake for any signs of illness.
3. Examine a fecal sample obtained by a colonic wash. Many snakes harbor internal parasites. If the owner will consent, a complete diagnostic workup including CBC/profile, C&S of the oral cavity (to check for infectious stomatitis), and whole body radiographs can be offered to screen for as many problems as possible. Unfortunately, many owners won't consent to these tests because of their expense, and a fecal test in an apparent "healthy" snake may be the only diagnostic procedure you can perform.
4. Treat any diseases that are present.
5. If the snake is obviously ill, force-feed it during the visit (see the discussion in chapter 5).

If the snake appears healthy and doesn't have any internal parasites, query the owner about the prey that has been given to the pet. Newly purchased pythons, for example, often should be left alone *without any handling* for 2–4 weeks so they can acclimate themselves to their new home. *Handling newly purchased snakes is a stress, and stress kills exotic pets!*

Newly imported snakes, snakes preparing to shed, and pregnant snakes will not feed. Some species of male snakes (some boas and pythons) refuse to feed during the breeding season, exhibiting a normal breeding season anorexia (2).

I suggest that owners try the following technique (3):

1. At night, introduce one or two live unweaned (fuzzy) rats. (These live animals are infants and will not harm the snake.) If this step fails, repeat it once a week at least two more times.
2. If the introduction of fuzzy rats fails, offer a freshly killed gerbil. Repeat this step once a week for 2 weeks.
3. If the gerbil offering fails, switch to the unweaned rats for 2 more weeks.
4. If no response is obtained, try a freshly killed, recently weaned rat. Next, try pinkie mice once a week for 2 weeks, followed by a freshly killed gerbil again for 2 weeks.

When trying this program, if prey isn't eaten within 24 hours, remove it and don't bother the snake until the next feeding.

As a rule, the snake should *not be handled* until it has started feeding. The client should *not* handle a snake within 72 hours after feeding, as it may induce a "feeding frenzy," causing the snake to strike the owner!

If the above steps fail, the brown bag method can be tried (3):

1. Take a brown grocery bag (paper bag) and punch a few holes in it.
2. Place the snake and a live unweaned rat in it, fold the top of the bag over, and staple shut. Leave overnight and check in the morning.
3. If this step fails, try it once weekly for 2 weeks.
4. If still unsuccessful, try the procedure with barely weaned gerbils or a freshly killed adult gerbil.

Yes, this process is a lot of work, and yes, owners have to be patient. Most snakes will eat at some point during these attempts. Occasionally, I will force-feed a snake to stimulate its gastrointestinal tract, and often I will use an appetite-stimulating dose of metronidazole (50–125 mg PO per snake given by stomach tube once) (4).

Eventually, most healthy snakes will eat; owners just need to experiment and find the right prey.

What size prey should a snake eat? As a rule, one prey item whose circumference is about equal to the snake's circumference at its widest point can be offered at each feeding. Of course, several items of smaller prey are also acceptable.

How often do snakes eat? Generally, the smaller snakes eat weekly or more often, whereas the larger ones eat every 1–4 weeks. This statement is extremely general; if an owner's snake eats only every few weeks, the owner will soon learn how often to feed it. For health reasons, uneaten prey should be removed from the cage within 24 hours.

Owners will probably have to kill the prey themselves, following one of several methods. The prey can be placed in a closed container with gas from a carbon dioxide (not monoxide) canister (dry ice is another form of this gas). Many pet owners place the prey (one at a time) in a paper bag and slam the bag against a table. The freshly stunned prey can then be offered immediately, or it can be killed by cutting its throat and freezing it for later thawing and feeding (cutting the throat of the stunned prey may induce the snake to eat the prey because of the presence of blood).

Many owners raise their own mice, gerbils, or rats instead of purchasing them from a pet store. This approach enables the owner to feed the rodents a nutritious diet, prior to feeding them to the snake. Finally, national dealers sell rodents to owners; the local herp club can offer names and addresses of some of these dealers.

This talk about killing prey and cutting throats might appear gruesome, but if an owner wants a snake as a pet it is a necessary step. If this process makes the client uncomfortable, he or she should consider another pet!

Fresh water in a crock that won't easily tip over should be available at all times. Snakes not only will drink from the water bowl but will often bathe in it as well (although it is perfectly acceptable to mist the python a few times a week as well). Make sure the water stays clean (many reptiles love to eliminate in their water dish).

■ BOX TURTLES

In the wild, box turtles are omnivorous, eating both plants and animals (plant and animal protein). As a result, they are relatively easy to feed. As with green iguanas, a diet consisting of only a few pieces of fruit and some crickets is totally inadequate (and is a cause of metabolic bone disease). Variety is the key, and the food must be chopped into small pieces so that the turtle can eat it.

The list of foods offered to iguanas is acceptable for box turtles as well. The main difference is that 50% of the box turtle's diet should be plant-based and 50% can be animal-based protein. Of the plant matter, most (80%) should be vegetable- or flower-based, and only 20% fruit-based. Even though turtles enjoy the sweetness of fruit, they are mineral-deficient compared with vegetables. Fruit should mainly be considered a treat.

Juvenile box turtles can be fed daily; adults can be fed daily or every other day. These recommendations are just guidelines, however, and many adult turtles will eat daily.

Fresh water in a shallow dish that won't easily tip over should be available at all times. Turtles not only will drink from the water bowl but will often bathe in it as well. Make sure the water stays clean (many reptiles love to eliminate in their water dish) and that the turtle can easily get into and out of the dish. Turtles can also be misted daily to keep them hydrated. Alternatively, many box turtles enjoy a daily swim in warm water (a shallow dish, sink, or tub works well), as long as the owner makes sure that the turtle does not drown.

In summary, variety is the key in feeding these reptiles. Don't let turtles get "hooked" on just one or two favorite items. Feed many items in small portions. Make sure the food is the right size for the turtle: smaller pets need their food finely chopped. As with all pets, fresh vegetables are preferred, frozen is second best, and canned is least desirable. Make up about a week's worth of the diet, and refrigerate or freeze the rest for convenience.

■ REFERENCES

1. Messonnier SP. Exotic Pets: A veterinary guide for owners. Plano, Texas: Wordware, 1995.
2. Boyer T. Breeding season anorexia in male snakes. Bull of ARAV 3:6.
3. De Vosjoli P. The general care and maintenance of ball pythons. Lakeside: Advanced Vivarium Series, 1990:11–14.
4. Frye F. Reptile care: An atlas of diseases and treatments, vols. I and II. Neptune City, NJ: TFH, 1991.

Clinical Procedures

▼   ▼   ▼   ▼   ▼   ▼   ▼   ▼

5

I N DIAGNOSING and treating reptiles, a veterinarian often has to perform certain procedures to obtain a diagnostic specimen or to carry out proper treatment. Ideally, the best way to learn these procedures is with "hands-on" guidance from a competent source. The following descriptions of the most frequently performed procedures can aid in your understanding of the techniques involved. It is strongly recommended that you attend a wet lab at a convention or work with an experienced veterinarian to learn these techniques.

■ COLONIC/CLOACAL WASH

Unlike the situation in mammals, a fecal flotation or smear is often inadequate for evaluating internal parasites in reptiles. Generally, the fecal material is solid and somewhat dry, especially in snakes. Protozoa, which are commonly diagnosed in reptiles, can't be detected in a dry sample. In contrast, nematodes can often be diagnosed with a *fresh* fecal sample. Whenever a fresh fecal sample is available, it is recommended that you use it along with material obtained from a colonic wash.

To evaluate a fecal sample, a colonic wash must be performed (if difficulty is encountered entering the colon, a cloacal wash can be performed instead, although the chance of a correct diagnosis is greater with a colonic wash). This technique will enable you to collect a fresh sample that can be directly examined via a microscope. The procedure is similar to an enema, except that the material is aspirated from the cloaca or colon and saved for examination (Fig. 5.1).

For snakes (1): An appropriately sized small red rubber feeding tube or tom cat catheter is used for the colonic wash. The tube is

▼

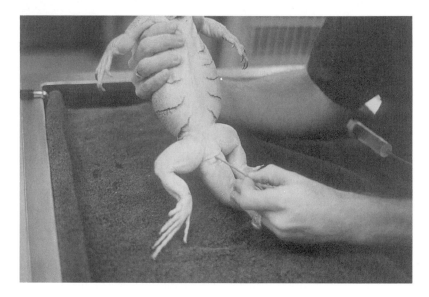

Fig. 5.1 *Inserting a red rubber feeding tube for a colonic wash in an iguana.*

lubricated with a water-soluble lubricant and *gently* inserted into the cloaca. Try to guide the tube into the colon via the ventral cloacal opening. Hold the snake with its ventrum upward and pinch off the ventral part of the cloaca as the tube is passed toward the cloacal opening. When the tube enters the colon, it will pass easily; if resistance is felt, the tube is pressing against the dead-end pouch of the cloaca. The tube is passed several inches into the colon, depending upon the size of the snake. Saline, approximately 2–6 mL per snake, is flushed and then aspirated. A colonic wash is preferable, but a cloacal wash will suffice if the tube cannot be guided into the colon. The aspirated material is then directly examined for parasite eggs (no flotation is needed).

The procedure is similar for other reptiles.

■ PER-CLOACAL DEWORMING

An alternative tehnique for deworming has been described in tortoises. Fenbendazole (Panacur 100 mg/mL) is administered per-cloacally to tortoises infected with oxyurids. The tortoise is placed in dorsal recumbency and the tip of a lubricated TB syringe gently inserted into the cloaca, with manual pressure applied circumferentially around the cloaca to prevent leakage of medication. Expulsion of oxyurids occurs immediately and for 2–3 days following the procedure; fecal flotations at 2 and 4 weeks after deworming failed to reveal ova. If possible, an attempt can be made to pass a red rubber catheter into the colon to prevent inadvertent passage of medication into the bladder. Per-cloacal administration of fenbendazole to tortoises or other species of reptiles may be an acceptable alternative to oral administration if this route of administration proves difficult or if several oral dewormings fail to eliminate the infection (2).

■ OROPHARYNGEAL/TRACHEAL WASH/SWAB (3,4)

A swab or wash of the oropharynx or trachea is often indicated in coughing or wheezing reptile patients. The throat or proximal trachea can be swabbed with a sterile cotton swab; the material can be evaluated cytologically or used for a culture and sensitivity. For a deeper specimen, a tracheal wash can be performed. Depending upon the size of the pet, 0.3–3.0 mL of warm, sterile saline is injected into the trachea through a sterile tom cat catheter and aspirated. The material can then be examined with a direct wet mount, a gram stain, or a culture and sensitivity test. Keep in mind that the normal oral flora is gram-negative, and the value of a gram stain is questionable unless fungal organisms, neoplastic cells, parasite ova, or a large amount of gram-positive organisms are identified.

■ FORCE FEEDING (3)

It is not uncommon for sick reptiles to be anorectic. Maintaining a positive nitrogen balance is critical; if the animal will not eat voluntarily, it must be force-fed. Reptiles should be rehydrated prior to force feeding.

Compared with dogs and cats, passing a gastric tube is easy in most reptiles because of the anatomy of the oral cavity. Especially in snakes, it is almost impossible to pass the tube into the "wrong" hole. Unlike mammals, the glottis is closed in the resting state in reptiles, making inadvertent intubation highly unlikely (3).

In general, a red rubber feeding tube of the appropriate size is lubricated and passed through the esophagus and into the stomach

(Fig. 5.2). The feeding material is introduced into the tube; at the completion of the feeding, the syringe is disconnected from the tube and a finger is placed over the end of the tube as it is withdrawn from the oral cavity. Stomach volume is estimated at 2% of body weight, or 20 mL/kg (5).

For snakes: The stomach is located at the junction of the second and third quarters of the snake's body. The tube is passed into the stomach by passing it at least half of the body length, which is fairly easy in small snakes. In longer snakes, the tube may not reach the stomach. In this case, an esophageal feeding occurs, which is also acceptable (1).

For iguanas: Measure the distance from the nose to the last rib. Open the mouth; note (and avoid) the trachea. An appropriate speculum (for example, a plastic syringe case) is used to hold the mouth open. The feeding tube is passed along the premeasured distance through the esophagus into the stomach. Alternatively, in small iguanas (less than 100 g), a 1 mL TB syringe without a needle can be used for force feeding. The syringe is passed through the esophagus into

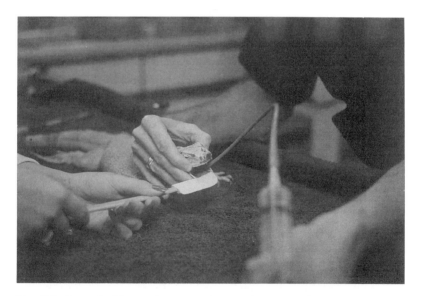

Fig. 5.2 *Force-feeding an iguana using a rubber spatula and red rubber feeding tube. A gruel of Emeraid II is used as the diet.*

the stomach while slowly twirling the syringe. It is passed one-third of the distance from the front legs to the rear legs to arrive in the stomach (6).

For turtles: Gently extend the neck and hold the turtle vertically. Measure the distance from the center of the plastron (where the stomach lies) to the front of the maxilla with the neck extended. Gently open the mouth and insert a speculum (a paper clip is used for small turtles; small mouth specula or hemostats also work). Pass the lubricated tube down the esophagus and into the stomach. Avoid the glottis at the base of the tongue. Keep the turtle vertical for 1 minute after feeding (7).

Some box turtles and iguanas will eat without tube feeding if the food is placed into the oral cavity with a syringe. Your choice of feeding technique depends upon the severity of the condition and the pet.

If regular force feeding is needed, an esophagostomy tube is easily placed and may be preferable to repeated force feedings if the animal is easily stressed (see below).

■ DIETS

For iguanas and box turtles: I mix 1 part Emeraid II diluted with 1–3 parts of warm water fresh at each feeding. The empirical dosage is 2.5 mL/100 g s.i.d.–t.i.d. Another option (for green iguanas) is to mix 1 part of alfalfa pellets with 2 parts of warm water and feed this mixture at 20 mL/kg q.o.d. for iguanas over 50 g of body weight. Make sure pets are adequately hydrated (through the use of oral or intracoelomic fluid administration) prior to force feeding (6).

Many veterinarians believe that feeding daily or one or two times a week is sufficient due to the slower gastrointestinal transit times in reptiles (3,6). I feel that as a rule slight overfeeding is preferable to underfeeding, and err on that side. Be careful that the stomach is emptied between feedings to avoid bloating or fermentation of the gastric contents. As more research is performed, an optimal feeding regimen should become available.

For snakes: I mix Emeraid II, 1–3 parts of warm water, and enough turkey baby food to make a slurry. This mixture is fed at a dosage of 10–20 mL/ft of snake (2.5–5.0 mL/100 g, or approximately

10–20 mL/lb). Empirically, I feed at least as often as the snake normally eats (usually every 1–4 weeks), and sometimes more often. Another acceptable diet is a slurry made with beaten raw eggs and meat-based baby food, fed in the same amounts as mentioned above (3).

It is important that snakes not be handled if at all possible for at least 48–72 hours postprandially; vomiting may result, and complete digestion takes 3–4 days (3). Treatments that need to be given postprandially should be performed quickly and with minimal stress to the patient.

Care must be used when feeding herbivorous reptiles as the intestinal microflora can be disrupted if large amounts of highly concentrated and fermentable carbohydrates are consumed. Occasionally, the microflora are disrupted when using antibiotics, especially oral doses. Gavage feeding with fecal material from disease-free reptiles can help reestablish normal microflora.

■ REHYDRATION

Water soaks: Turtles and tortoises can absorb water through their cloacal openings (7,8). All hospitalized reptiles can benefit from several (t.i.d.) soaks in warm water (80–90 °F) in addition to injectable rehydration therapy. These soaks not only aid in rehydration but also encourage elimination, provide a source of warmth, and simulate a natural activity for the pet (Fig. 5.3). The soaks last 5–15 minutes; warm water is added as the existing water begins to cool. Care must be taken to ensure the animals do not drown in the water bath.

Intracoelomic injections: The intracoelomic (turtles, snakes, and iguanas) and epicoelomic (turtles) routes are used for fluid therapy, as well as occasionally an injectable medication (such as calcium for metabolic bone disease in iguanas). In making injections, advance the needle just far enough to enter the coelomic cavity without penetrating the viscera. Needle lengths and gauges vary according to the size of the pet. For most small iguanas and turtles, as well as most snakes of any size, a 1-in. needle suffices. Typically, I use needles that range from 22 to 25 gauge in size. Lactated Ringer's, PSS, or "Reptile Ringer's" (see Appendix I) can be used at a dose of 15–25 mL/kg q24 hours for maintenance; additional fluid is given as based on estimated dehydration. Warming of the fluid may be needed (3).

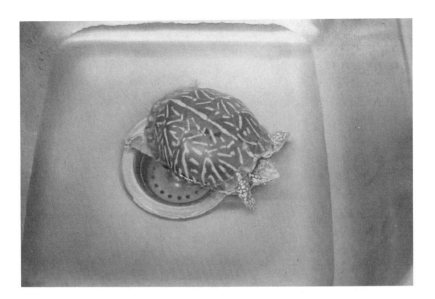

Fig. 5.3 *Soaking hospitalized reptile patients in a warm-water bath is extremely helpful to their recovery.*

For iguanas: Inject the fluid into the caudal paralumbar abdominal space (see Fig. 5.4), which is located in front of the femur, about one-third of the distance ventrally from the dorsal midline (7). The animal struggles less if the injection is given in this location while the pet is in a normal "sitting" posture. Injections can be given in the caudal ventral abdomen with the iguana placed on its back; however, the iguana seems to struggle more in this position. Subcutaneous injections are given in the dorsal flank, axillary, or interscapular area. Although some authors call this procedure an intraperitoneal injection, technically this name is incorrect because iguanas lack a diaphragm and, therefore, a peritoneal cavity.

For snakes: An injection is made anywhere along the ventrum of the snake. Ideally, the needle passes between—and not through—the scales. Insert the needle only far enough to penetrate the coelomic membrane and enter the body cavity (3). Alternatively, SQ fluids can be given in the lateral sinus, which is located at the junction between the epaxial muscles and the ribs (3).

For turtles: Intracoelomic injections are made just cranial to the hindlimb. An epicoelomic injection is approached by directing the

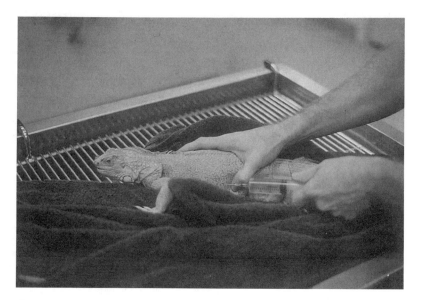

Fig. 5.4 *An intracoelomic injection of fluids is used for rehydration in an iguana.*

needle caudally just ventral to the shoulder joint (pectoral girdle) and dorsal to the plastron; the needle is passed through the pectoral muscles into the epicoelomic space, and directed toward the contralateral hindlimb. Epicoelomic injections are preferred if the turtle is suffering from severe respiratory disease (pneumonia) (10). Epicoelomic injections also avoid possible lung laceration (which may occur with intracoelomic injections) and do not compromise lung space within the shell cavity (5).

■ ESOPHAGOSTOMY/PHARYNGOSTOMY

If a feeding tube needs to be placed, an esophagostomy will be required. With the animal anesthetized (and intubated if desired), a small pair of curved mosquito hemostats is introduced through the oral cavity and into the esophagus. The tips of the hemostat are gently pressed against the wall of the esophagus until a slight bulge becomes visible through the skin externally. A tiny incision is made between the scales, through the skin and soft tissue, and into the esophagus. An appropriately sized red rubber feeding tube is placed through this incision and grasped intraorally with the hemostats. The tip of the tube is then directed aborally and into the stomach. The external part of the tube is sutured to the skin. Excess tube is trimmed and discarded; the remaining tip of the tube is capped. This technique is useful for iguanas and snakes; it is impractical in turtles as they retract their heads into their shells (3).

■ VENIPUNCTURE (3,10)

Several venipuncture methods are available (my method of choice is highlighted with an asterisk). Only small volumes of blood are needed to run most tests (green-top lithium heparin tubes can be used to run a CBC and biochemical profiles on small volumes of blood). You may find it helpful to contact your laboratory of choice to determine the exact specimens needed.

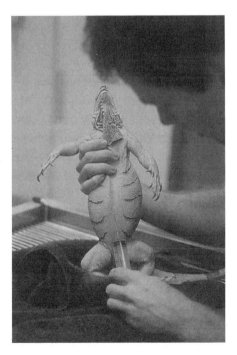

Fig. 5.5 *Venipuncture in an iguana using the ventral (central) midline vein.*

For iguanas:

1. Ventral (central) midline vein (Fig. 5.5)
2. Toenail
3. Ventral caudal (tail) vein*
4. Cardiac tap (last resort)

For snakes:

1. Cardiac puncture (many veterinarians use this option as their site of choice; others prefer another site as a first choice)*
2. Ventral caudal (tail) vein
3. Dorsal/ventral buccal veins

For turtles:

1. Jugular vein*
2. Axillary vein
3. Toenail
4. Cardiac tap (requires a hole drilled through plastron)
5. Posterior occipital venous sinus

■ SEX DETERMINATION

Many owners inquire as to the sex of their reptile pet. There are several methods of sex determination.

For snakes: Metal sexing probes can be used to probe the caudal cloacal area. I find 3 1/2 in. Sovereign tom cat catheters useful. The probe or catheter is lubricated with a water-soluble lubricant; the snake is slightly flexed dorsally and the probe or catheter gently directed caudally from the cloaca along the lateral borders (walls) of the cloaca. In female snakes, the probe or catheter will advance only 2–3 scales. In males, the probe or catheter will advance into the hemipenile sheaths—a distance of 8–16 subcaudal scales (1).

In iguanas: The same probing technique can be used. In larger iguanas, sex determination can be made visually. Male iguanas have much larger femoral pores located along the medial femurs (see Fig. 5.6) than female iguanas. This method is most accurate in iguanas with a snout-to-vent length greater than 20 cm.

In box turtles: The female's cloaca is closer to the base of a short, stubby tail. Her irises are yellow to red–brown. Male box turtles have

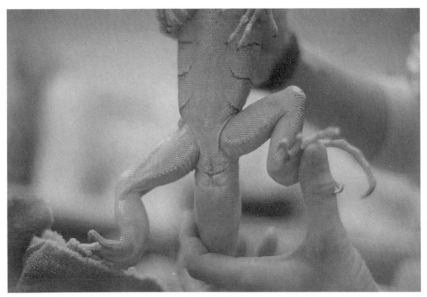

Fig. 5.6 *Large femoral pores on the medial aspects of the thigh indicate that this iguana is an adult male.*

longer, thicker tails, the cloaca is further from the base, the irises are bright red, and the claws of the inner hind toes are thicker and hooked medially. Plastron concavity is not reliable in sexing box turtles (7).

■ ANESTHESIA (12,13,14)

Several regimens are available, and each practitioner will have a favorite drug or combination of drugs. I prefer isoflurane because of its relatively quick induction and recovery with few side effects. Induction is accomplished via masking (iguanas) or by chamber (iguanas, snakes, and turtles). Once the anesthetic is induced, maintenance takes place by mask or endotracheal tubes. Masks can be custom-made from syringe cases to fit a variety of pets.

I use the anesthetic chamber to induce isoflurance in this fashion (see Fig. 5.7). After the pet is placed into the chamber, I use 2 liters of oxygen with 2% isoflurane. After 1–2 minutes, the concentration of isoflurane is increased 1% per minute, until a 5% concentration is reached. The pets seem to struggle less (if at all) using this method as compared with using the straight 5% concentration immediately.

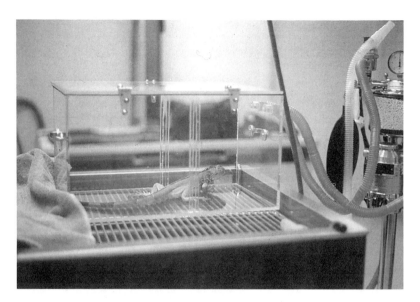

Fig. 5.7 *Inducing anesthesia with isoflurane using an anesthetic induction chamber.*

Maintenance involves 1–3% isoflurane using a mask (short procedures; see Fig. 5.8) or intubation.

Reptiles can undergo prolonged apnea, although I have not had a problem with inhalant induction. Some practitioners premedicate with an injectable anesthetic (ketamine + / − atropine) and then intubate 30 minutes later. Regardless of the induction method, intubation can usually be easily accomplished once the righting reflex is lost.

For intubation, tubes can be fashioned from polypropylene tom cat urinary catheters or red rubber feeding tubes; cuffed infant tubes and Cole tubes also work well. The trachea of lizards and snakes is composed of incomplete tracheal rings with a dorsal tracheal membrane; chelonians have complete tracheal rings. Chelonians have a very short trachea cranial to the bifurcation; care must be taken not to intubate a bronchus. The lungs of reptiles are structurally simpler than the lungs of mammals. The left lung is absent or vestigial in most snakes but is developed in boas and pythons. The right lung extends almost to the level of the vent. Lungs of reptiles are fragile, and care must be exercised when positive-pressure ventilation is performed.

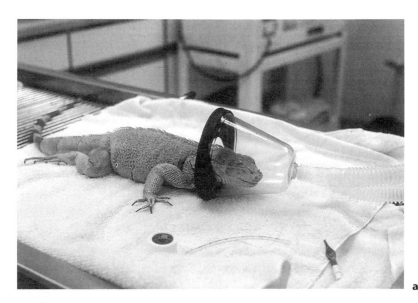

a

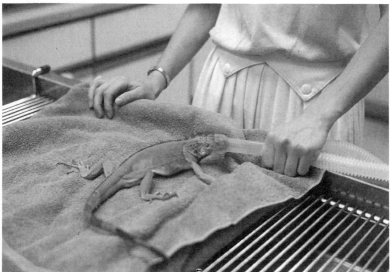

b

Fig. 5.8(a & b) *After induction, the iguana is maintained on anesthetic using a mask. A syringe case adapted for use as a mask works well for smaller pets.*

The glottis of reptiles remains closed between breaths and opens for respiration. Muscles of the abdomen and trunk work with the intercostal muscles for breathing as reptiles do not possess a diaphragm (chelonians, which do not have intercostal muscles, also use changes in the position of abdominal and thoracic viscera for respiration). In addition, smooth muscles present within the walls of the lungs assist in respiration.

Reptiles have a remarkable ability to resist hypoxia. Every attempt should be made to revive reptiles that appear "dead."

Non-rebreathing systems are recommended on reptiles under 10 kg; I have, however, used rebreathing systems without problems. The maintenance dose of isoflurane is 1–3% with oxygen flow at 1 liter/min.

When possible, sick animals should be stabilized prior to anesthetic procedures; supplemental heat can be supplied as needed. Reptiles should be kept at 75–85 °F or at the warmer end of their thermoneutral zone during induction, surgery, and the postoperative recovery period. Excessive heat should be avoided as it increases tissue oxygen demand. Doxapram (Dopram-V, 20 mg/mL, Ft. Dodge) at 0.25 mL/kg IV can stimulate respiration if needed.

Monitoring anesthetic depth is more difficult in reptiles than in mammals. During anesthesia, relaxation progresses from cranial to caudal and motor function returns from caudal to cranial. The righting reflex is the first reflex lost as a reptile becomes anesthetized. Failure to move the tail or foot when pinched indicates a surgical plane of anesthesia. The corneal reflex (which is not present in snakes because of their spectacles) is present at a surgical plane of anesthesia but is lost when the patient is too deep into the anesthetic condition. Assisted ventilation may be needed at a surgical plane of anesthesia, although I have safely maintained reptiles on gas anesthesia with a mask for procedures lasting up to 2 hours without problems. It is probably wise to consider intubation for any reptile that will be anesthetized for longer than 30–60 minutes.

Constant monitoring and adjustment of anesthetic concentration are often needed because inhalation anesthesia is not usually as smooth in reptiles as in mammals. An EKG can be used even though the QRS patterns are generally inverted and slurred. A Doppler flow monitor can also be used as an audible measure of heart activity. Stethoscopy is difficult in reptiles.

Injectable Regimens

Atropine: Premedication with atropine (0.01–0.04 mg/kg SQ, IM) (13) or glycopyrrolate (0.01 mg/kg SQ, IM) (13) at 30 minutes prior to induction is recommended to reduce oral and upper respiratory secretions that may block small endotracheal tubes.

Ketamine: Ketamine is useful for minor surgical procedures (e.g., suturing a wound) or as a premedicant for invasive procedures. It is injected in the following dosages:

Snakes: 30–60 mg/kg SQ, IM (13)
Iguanas: 30–40 mg/kg SQ, IM (13)
Turtles: 40–60 mg/kg SQ, IM (13)

Ideally, the injection should be made in the cranial half of the pet to avoid the renal portal system. The lower dosages produce tranquilization; the higher dosages will produce deeper sedation and perhaps apnea. Some movement may occur even with higher dosages. Larger reptiles with slower metabolisms will require lower dosages than smaller reptiles. Sedation is seen within 10–30 minutes; recovery can take hours or days (especially at higher dosages; prolonged recovery is common in turtles) but usually is complete within 3–4 hours. Iguanas recover more rapidly than snakes, and turtles recover slowly. Some authors advise against using ketamine in lizards due to possible fatalities.

Telazol: 20–40 mg/kg IM in iguanas and snakes, 5–15 mg/kg in turtles (13). *Use of Telazol is contraindicated if ivermectin has been used or will be used within 10 days due to zolazepam fraction.* Use a lower dose for shorter procedures. The time between the initial injection and arousal is approximately 1 hour.

Succinylcholine: 0.5–1.0 mg/kg IM in turtles, 0.75–1.0 mg/kg IM in iguanas (13). An effect is seen within 4–6 minutes; it lasts 20 minutes. Succinylcholine is used for short-term restraint in chelonians to allow the head and limbs to be withdrawn from the shell. If higher dosages are used, respiration may need to be mechanically assisted. Occasionally, a chelonian will rigidly extend its limbs for

1–2 minutes after the injection; respiration should be monitored and assisted if needed. Complete recovery is seen within 45–60 minutes. Succinylcholine provides no anesthesia or analgesia.

Hypothermia

Hypothermia is *not recommended* as no anesthesia is produced. In addition, the immune system is depressed in this process.

■ RADIOLOGY

Each practitioner has a favorite film–screen combination. Most veterinarians recommend film and screen combinations that give the best detail and allow for short exposure times. Rare earth screen and film combinations fit this need. I use the same rare earth films and screens for reptiles as I do for canine, feline, and avian radiology. At least two views should be taken. My standard views for chelonians are a DV, standing lateral using a horizontal beam, and a cranial–caudal (skyline) view. These options allow excellent visualization of the viscera, especially the lung fields. An acceptable technique is 5 mAs (300 mA, 1/60 sec or 100 mA, 1/20 sec) with a kVp of 50–75 depending upon the size of the pet. Some radiologists suggest decreasing the focal spot-film distance to 30 in. and decreasing mA by one-half for small exotic pets. Radiographs can often be prepared on an animal while it is awake; sedation may be used if needed. A reference book should be consulted for more information on this topic and on comparative anatomy.

■ REFERENCES

1. Russo ER. Diagnosis and treatment of lumps and bumps in snakes. Compend Contin Educ Pract Vet, August 1987; 9:795–802.
2. Innis C. Per-cloacal worming in tortoises. Bull of ARAV; 5:4.
3. Frye F. Reptile care: An atlas of diseases and treatments, vols. I and II. Neptune City, NJ: TFH, 1991.
4. Anderson N. Husbandry and clinical evaluation of *Iguana iguana*. Compend Contin Educ Pract Vet, August 1991; 13:1265–1269.
5. Boyer T. Emergency care of reptiles. Seminars in avian and exotic pet medicine, October 1994; 3:210–216.
6. Boyer T. Common problems and treatment of green iguanas (*Iguana iguana*). Bull of ARAV, 1991; Premiere Issue: 8–11.

7. Boyer T. Common problems of box turtles in captivity. Bull of ARAV 2:9–16.

8. Boyer D, Boyer T. Tortoise care. Bull of ARAV 4:16–27.

9. Jenkins J. Medical management of reptile patients. Compend Contin Educ Pract Vet, June 1991; 13:980–988.

10. Rosskopf WJ, *et al.* A practical method of performing venipuncture in snakes. VM/SAC, May 1982:820–821.

11. Rodda GH. Sexing *Iguana iguana.* Bull Chicago Herp Soc, 1991; 26:173–175.

12. Anderson N. Diseases of *Iguana iguana.* Compend Contin Educ Pract Vet, October 1992; 14:1335–1342.

13. Boyer T. Clinical anesthesia of reptiles. Bull of ARAV 2:10–12.

14. Bennett RA. Reptile anesthesia. In: Current veterinary therapy XII. Philadelphia: WB Saunders, 1995:1349–1353.

Common Diseases of Reptiles

▼   ▼   ▼   ▼   ▼   ▼   ▼   ▼

As WITH many exotic pets, the most common reptile diseases occur as a result of owner misinformation. Improper feeding and improper environment (housing) contribute to most of the problems seen by reptile veterinarians. Even many infections are secondary to poor diet and environment as sources of disease. Therefore, with the proper knowledge some of the diseases seen frequently in pet reptiles can be prevented.

With regard to infectious diseases, you should keep in mind that few medications are approved specifically for use in reptiles. Dosages of medications have often been extrapolated from other species or determined from clinical experience rather than exhaustive biomedical research. Most of the medications require off-label usage.

Unlike other pets, reptiles often require longer treatment periods, especially for infectious diseases. It is recommended to treat reptile infections for at least 2–3 weeks with appropriate antimicrobial therapy. Increasing the environmental temperature to the upper extreme of the pet's comfort zone increases the chance for cure. The cell-mediated and humoral immune responses are temperature-dependent; the immune response is maximized and the pathogenicity of many infectious organisms is decreased as the ambient temperature is increased. When what appear to be simple bacterial infections do not resolve, consider other possibilities (e.g., concurrent nutritional or environmental deficiencies, mycobacterial infection, underlying parasitic infection, viral infection, anaerobic bacterial infections).

Diseases and Treatment of Iguanas

▼   ▼   ▼   ▼   ▼   ▼   ▼   ▼

■ COMMONLY SEEN CONDITIONS

Metabolic Bone Disease

Metabolic bone disease—also called nutritional osteodystrophy, nutritional secondary hyperparathyroidism, or rubber jaw—is probably *the* most common disease of iguanas. The condition typically results from a lack of calcium and/or vitamin D_3 in the diet. Increased dietary phosphorus, primary renal or hepatic disease, or thyroid or parathyroid disease can also cause metabolic bone disease (1).

Even though the blood calcium level usually remains normal, the animal can show signs of illness. Early signs include swelling of the mandibles (see Fig. 6.1a); later, swelling of the limbs, usually the rear legs, is seen (see Fig. 6.1b). Many owners often mistake this swelling for increased muscularity, despite the fact that the iguana may be losing weight and actually appears thin. Later in the course of the disease, weakness, lethargy, and anorexia become evident. Pathologic fractures can occur due to cortical bone thinning, and paralysis may result if the spine is fractured and the spinal cord is severed. Hypocalcemic tetany may be manifested by muscle twitching. A plantigrade or palmigrade stance (walking on the hocks or wrist) may also appear as a sign of weakness. With metabolic bone disease, any combination of these symptoms is possible.

In my experience, if the iguana is still eating and active, the prognosis for recovery is good to excellent. The first step in treatment is a complete physical examination. Often, sick animals also have infectious stomatitis, septicemia, and infection with internal parasites. A good examination can provide a wealth of prognostic information.

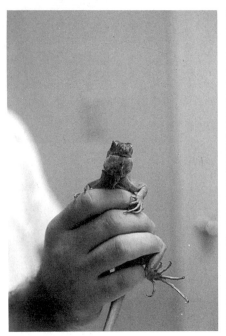
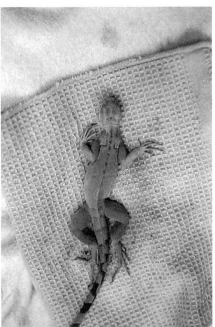

a   b

Fig. 6.1(a & b) *Mandibular swelling and swelling of the limbs are classic symptoms of metabolic bone disease in iguanas.*

Radiographs are not usually needed for diagnosis of metabolic bone disease unless the iguana does not respond to conventional treatment. Radiographs can reveal other pathology of co-existing problems, however, so some clinicians may recommend them. Individuals with parasites, infectious stomatitis, or other problems need these conditions addressed in addition to the metabolic bone disease.

Iguanas that are still active and eating can usually be treated at home. Either oral or injectable calcium can be administered by the owner if the decision is made to use this treatment option. If calcitonin is the preferred treatment, oral calcium is administered at home by the owner and the calcitonin is administered in the hospital. Calcium injections (see the "Treatment" section) are given intracoelomically* by the owner (most owners can easily be taught to perform this procedure). Vitamins are also used as part of the treatment regimen. The owner should be instructed to supply ultraviolet light

---

*Intracoelomic is the correct term because iguanas lack a diaphragm and, therefore, a peritoneal cavity. Some authors use the term *intraperitoneal* interchangably with intracoelomic.

(UV-B light in the 290–320 nm range) and *slowly* begin changing the diet. The easiest way to accomplish this goal is by adding a small amount of a balanced vegetable mixture (see chapter 4) and decreasing the regular diet by about 10% per week. The diet must eventually be changed; the iguana may refuse to eat the new diet at first, but it's more important for the pet to eat a bad diet than nothing at all. The treatment with injectable calcium and UV light may allow the iguana to improve despite the bad diet. Recovery, if it occurs, should be seen after 4–6 weeks of injections.

Owners are instructed to remove all objects from the cage except the food and water bowls. The bones of pets with this disease are very fragile and can easily fracture if the iguana falls off a basking area or if a tree limb falls onto the pet.

Iguanas that are lethargic and anorectic have a guarded prognosis, but treatment should always be offered to the owner. In my experience, 25–50% of seriously ill iguanas may respond to aggressive therapy. Such animals require hospitalization in which they are placed in an incubator and given intracoelomic fluids. Force feeding is used to overcome the catabolic state and stimulate appetite. If improvement occurs, it usually takes place within 2–3 days of intensive care.

Treatment (Mild Cases)

Currently there are two options for treatment of metabolic bone disease. Option I uses either oral or injectable (or both) calcium and has been the standard treatment for metabolic bone disease for many years. Option II involving 3 weekly visits, utilizes oral calcium and calcitonin injections and is a newer suggested protocol. I have used both treatment options with equal success but currently prefer Option II, as it allows closer monitoring of the pets because of the necessity for repeated office visits.

Option I
1.   Several regimens for calcium injections exist:
     • 10% calcium gluconate, 100 mg/mL, 500 mg/kg intracoelomically weekly for 4–6 weeks* (1,2); or Calphosan

*Note that 4–6 weeks is an arbitrary period during which most pets respond to treatment. If the iguana is responding but not yet "cured," the treatment can be extended as needed.

0.5–1.0 mL/(50–100 mg/kg IM weekly for 4–6 weeks* (3) Alternatively, oral calcium (Neo-Calglucon at 1 mL/kg b.i.d. for 2–3 months) can be used instead of injectable calcium. For iguanas that have severe limb or mandibular swelling or that exhibit signs of tetany, an injection of calcium gluconate (500 mg/kg) can be given and then the pet can be started on oral calcium.

2. Dietary correction.
3. UV light.
4. Remove branches and other objects that might injure the pet.
5. B-complex vitamin injection: 0.25–0.50 mL/kg (once is usually adequate) (4).
6. Injacom-100: Dose at 100 IU vitamin D_3/kg SQ, two doses one week apart (5).
7. Mineral supplementation: Osteoform tablets are acceptable; dose at 200 IU D_3/kg/week (1). The tablets should be crushed and the correct amount sprinkled on the food weekly. After 2–4 months, you can switch to a supplement containing only calcium to avoid hypervitaminosis D. As a rule, a daily sprinkling of a calcium supplement is adequate. The amount to sprinkle on the food is equivalent to the *light* salting a person would give to his or her own food.
8. Vitamin supplementation: A light sprinkling 1–2 times per week of a good avian or reptile vitamin or one crushed Centrum tablet is adequate.
9. If no improvement occurs after 4–6 weeks of therapy, reevaluate the iguana for other conditions (e.g., parasites, stomatitis) or a different diagnosis. Radiographs may help to evaluate

*Note that the dosages of calcium for the two regimens listed (intracoelomic calcium and intramuscular calcium) are vastly different. The dosage of intracoelomic calcium gluconate is 500 mg/kg and the dosage of intramuscular Calphosan is 50–100 mg/kg. I have used both regimens without side effects and find them successful in the treatment of metabolic bone disease. Because of the large volume of calcium gluconate needed (at this dosage) for larger lizards, I usually apply the intracoelomic regimen in smaller iguanas and the intramuscular Calphosan in larger iguanas and other lizards. These dosages have been referenced from the literature (see Appendix I), which has not offered a discussion on why the mg/kg dosages differ vastly. It may be that the "correct" dosage of calcium (regardless of the form of calcium) for treating metabolic bone disease is 50–100 mg/kg, but this idea remains to be proven.

bone density. Ensure that the owner is adequately injecting the calcium at home. You may consider increasing the calcium dosage by 1.5–2.0 times the recommended dosage. Calcitonin may be needed as part of the therapy (see below).

Option II (5)

1. Start calcium glubionate (Neo–Calglucon syrup, USP) at 1 mL/kg PO q12h on the first visit. 10% Calcium gluconate (100 mg/kg IM q6h prn for up to 24 hours) can be given if hypocalcemic tetany is present. (I often give an initial ICe injection of 10% calcium gluconate at 500 mg/kg at the first visit if tetany or severe mandibular or limb swelling is present.) The Neocalglucon can be continued for more than a year or even for the life of the iguana. After stabilization (usually 2–3 months), you may switch to an s.i.d. regimen.
2. Give Injacom-100 (dosed at 1000 IU vitamin D_3/kg) IM once weekly for two treatments. (first and second week)
3. If the iguana is normocalcemic, give calcitonin (Calcimar, 200 IU/mL) at 50 IU/kg IM once weekly at the week 2 and 3 visits. (If serum calcium levels are unknown, no problem should be encountered with using the calcitonin as long as the Neocalglucon has been given as directed.)

Treatment (Severe Cases, Anorexia/Lethargy)

1. Give intracoelomic or SQ injections of fluids at 15–25 mL/kg/day (1–3% of body weight/day) for maintenance, and more if dehydrated as calculated (2).
2. Incubation at 90–100 °F in the hospital incubator.
3. Force feeding with Emeraid II at 10–15 mL/500 g s.i.d.–b.i.d. of reconstituted product after rehydration of the iguana.
4. Warm water soaks b.i.d.–q.i.d.

While the diagnosis of metabolic bone disease is usually straightforward (history of incorrect diet, no UV light provided), I have seen several lizards that responded to treatment for metabolic bone disease (calcium injections) despite the appearance of an adequate diet and environment. These animals were offered a variety of vegetables and were supplied a UV light. In some instances, the UV light had "aged" (i.e., it was older than 6 months); as noted in chapter 3, UV lights should be replaced every 6–12 months because the UV output decreases with age. Owners of these lizards presumed their pets were receiving adequate UV light, when in fact that may not have been true. The symptoms seen in these pets, which were supposedly offered a variety of vegetables and had exposure to (aged) UV light, were nonspecific and included anorexia, lethargy, weakness, and in a few cases muscle tremors (symptoms possibly related to hypocalcemia). Because metabolic bone disease is the most common disease in iguanas, it should be suspected in any sick iguana, even those without the characteristic swelling of the mandibles and rear limbs and in those supposedly on an adequate plane of nutrition. Diagnosis can be made through radiology, serum calcium levels, or response to treatment in cases where owners will not give permission for diagnostic testing.

Infectious Stomatitis

Infectious stomatitis is more commonly known as "mouth rot." The disease is almost always caused by bacteria. While many bacterial species are capable of causing the problem, *Pseudomonas* and *Aeromonas* are typically the culprits. Many doctors feel that this disease is always a secondary condition, as *Pseudomonas* and *Aeromonas* are often normally present in a reptile's environment and body.

Certainly a filthy environment contributes to this problem, but I have seen cases involving animals housed in what owners described as clean environments. Other stressors that can cause the disease include internal parasites, poor diet, improper environment and improper environmental temperature (low body temperature in any animal decreases the ability of the body's immune system to fight off infection; for the ectothermic reptiles, proper environmental temperature is critical to survival), shipping (e.g., when a pet is brought into an owner's home after purchase), too little or too much handling, a too humid or too dry cage, and almost any other stress. The stress isn't always identified, but the pet should undergo a thorough diagnostic workup (treat the pet, not the disease!).

Early symptoms that often go unnoticed by owners are petechial hemorrhages inside the oral cavity. These signs are often observed during a routine physical examination of an asymptomatic iguana or in the oral cavity of an iguana presented for another medical problem. Don't overlook these early lesions; begin treatment if they are detected. The later stages reveal a large amount of frothy, bubbly mucus or a "cottage cheese" type of exudate. Many animals in the later stages are also anorectic and lethargic.

Diagnosis of infectious stomatitis is fairly easy and is made by observation of the oral cavity. All obvious cases as well as suspected cases (where the amount or character of the mucus seems slightly abnormal or where only petechial hemorrhages are present) should be cultured. *Pseudomonas* and *Aeromonas* are found in many normal reptiles, so their presence on a culture doesn't always mean the pet has, or will develop, mouth rot. Any heavy growth on a culture, particularly in the presence of clinical signs or heavy growth of a single bacterial species, should probably be treated, however.

Treatment varies with the severity of the disease. As with any disease, pets that are lethargic and anorectic need hospitalization. During hospitalization, these severely ill patients are given fluids, kept warm in an incubator (90–100 °F), and force-fed.

While practitioners are awaiting culture results, iguanas are started on injectable antibiotics. The oral cavity is treated with a topical medication, such as dilute povidone–iodine solution, chlorhexidine solution, hydrogen peroxide, and/or Silvadene. Some practitioners report good success when using Maxi-Guard gel topically in addition to parenteral antibiotic therapy. Atropine injections can be used if the mucus is thick and tenacious; many veterinarians feel that atropine helps to thin the mucus and allow for easier removal by the animal's body (2). Vitamin B complex injections are given. Vitamin C injections also seem to be efficacious in many cases of stomatitis (2).

The prognosis of infectious stomatitis depends upon several factors. If the animal is still eating and active and no other diseases are detected, the prognosis is usually good. If signs are caught early when only petechial hemorrhages are seen, the prognosis is also very good. Animals that haven't eaten in several days or weeks, are weak and depressed, and have large amounts of mucus in their oral cavities are often septic and have a much poorer chance of recovery. Secondary problems, such as internal parasites, also need to be addressed. Once the animal has recovered, the diet is slowly corrected and the environment is changed.

Treatment (Mild Cases)

1. Culture and sensitivity test of oral cavity (possibly including anaerobic cultures).
2. Begin therapy with any of the following antibiotics pending C&S results: (see Formulary for an in-depth discussion).
   - Amikacin: 2.5 mg/kg SQ, IM every 72 hours for 5–7 treatments* (2,4)
   - Piperacillin: 200–400 mg/kg IM q24h* ** (4)
   - Cephalothin: 40–80 mg/kg dd b.i.d.* ** (2)
   - Trimethoprim–Sulfadiazine: 30 mg/kg SQ, IM q24h for 10–14 treatments* (4)
3. Oral therapy should include any of the following topical rinses:
   - Dilute chlorhexidine solution (0.25–0.50%) (2)
   - Dilute povidone–iodine solution (1%) (2)
   - Acetic acid (vinegar) (dilute to a 0.5% solution) (2)
   - Hydrogen peroxide (2)

   Rinses are given b.i.d.; the mouth is rinsed with plain water after the rinses are used. Alternating rinses (i.e., chlorhexidine day 1, peroxide day 2, acetic acid day 3, then repeat for the duration of treatment) may be helpful. I alternate rinses as follows: chlorhexidine followed by peroxide followed by tap water on day 1, chlorhexidine followed by vinegar followed by water on day 2. This regimen is repeated on subsequent days. The vinegar (acetic acid) produces an acid environment; the peroxide produces an oxygenated environment that is not conducive to anaerobic organisms. *Wear eye protection (goggles) and have clients do the same when rinsing the oral cavity!*
4. Topical Silvadene is applied after oral rinses.

Treatment (Severe Cases)

1. In addition to the treatment listed for mild cases, pets with severe cases of stomatitis need hospitalization with fluid therapy (15–25 mL/kg/day for maintenance), incubation (95–100 °F), and force feeding (see chapter 5).

* Any of these agents is a rational choice for first-time antibiotic selection. Save enrofloxacin for the more serious cases.
** Combine with amikacin.

2. In addition, you may want to use enrofloxacin $+/-$ amikacin as your initial antibiotic selection.
   - Enrofloxacin: 10 mg/kg IM q24h for 10–14 days (4,6)

Many veterinarians recommend parenteral fluids in any reptile receiving aminoglycosides, and to a lesser extent piperacillin and cephalosporins, to prevent renal damage (2).

For cases that don't respond to appropriate antimicrobial therapy, consider an anaerobic infection. Perform an anaerobic culture and treat with metronidazole, clindamycin, or tetracycline. Anaerobes may account for as much as 50% of bacterial infections in reptiles.

Respiratory Disease

Respiratory diseases may occur secondary to other conditions, such as improper diet, environment, or infectious stomatitis. Respiratory disease can be as mild as rhinitis or as severe as pneumonia; causative organisms include bacteria (most commonly), fungi, viruses, and parasites. Lack of a diaphragm prevents active coughing from the air-sac-like lungs of reptiles, and the mainstem bronchi and trachea enter the lungs more cranially than in mammals (2). These factors favor the retention of respiratory secretions in the lower airways; simple respiratory infections are more prone to developing into pneumonia than in mammals (2). Conversely, muscular anaerobiasis (glycolic respiration) is remarkable in reptiles; they can often survive respiratory infections that would prove fatal to animals lacking anaerobic respiratory capabilities (2).

Many "simple" respiratory infections in reptiles are actually signs of serious lower respiratory disease and may require aggressive treatment. While the prognosis for such infections is always guarded, many reptiles will survive *if* appropriate aggressive treatment is instituted. To be safe, any reptile that is anorectic and lethargic and has respiratory symptoms (e.g., sneezing, wheezing, mucopurulent nasal discharge, dyspnea, open-mouth breathing) should be presumed to have pneumonia until proved otherwise and treated aggressively. Many of these pets are gravely ill and hospitalization is essential. Hospitalized iguanas are kept in an incubator given fluids and force fed. Cultures (both aerobic and anaerobic, if needed) of the respiratory tract are taken, and a tracheal and colonic wash are performed to examine for parasites and other infectious organisms. Injectable antibiotics are given. Once the iguana begins to improve, the owner can continue antibiotic injections at home.

Iguanas that appear healthy and present with only mild signs of respiratory disease can be treated at home with vitamins and antibiotics if indicated.

Treatment

1. Maintain hydration with intracoelomic fluids (15–25 mL/kg/day for maintenance) (2).
2. Force-feed as needed.
3. Begin antibiotic therapy with the following, pending C&S results: (see Formulary for an in-depth discussion).)
    *   Amikacin: 2.5 mg/kg SQ, IM every 72 hours for 5–7 treatments* (2,4)
    *   Piperacillin: 200–400 mg/kg IM q24h* ** (4)
    *   Cephalothin: 40–80 mg/kg dd b.i.d.* ** (2)
    *   Trimethoprim–Sulfadiazine: 30 mg/kg SQ, IM q24h for 10–14 treatments* (4)

    You may want to use enrofloxacin (10 mg/kg IM q24h for 10–14 days [6,12]) +/− amikacin as your initial antibiotic selection.
4. Perform a tracheal wash, cytology, and culture and sensitivity test as needed.
5. Perform a fecal flotation.
6. Maintain a warm (95–100 °F) environment.
7. Nebulization using amikacin or gentamicin may be indicated. Regimens and dosages of medications follow those used with birds and mammals. Some veterinarians advocate adding a bronchodilator (Albuterol), cromalyn sodium, and/or acetylcysteine to the nebulizing solution.

---

* Any of these agents is a rational choice for first-time antibiotic selection. Save enrofloxacin for the more serious cases.
** Combine with amikacin.

8. Oxygen therapy as needed.
9. Furosemide (5 mg/kg IV, IM prn) can help reduce respiratory fluids; parenteral fluids should be used concurrently with diuretics (2).
10. Atropine (0.04 mg/kg PO, IV, IM, SQ prn) can help dry mucous membranes (2).

Anorexia/Constipation/Regurgitation Syndrome

Anorexia/constipation/regurgitation syndrome (3) is an ill-defined condition that is usually seen in iguanas that fail to adapt to captivity. Often the iguana has had a recent change in owner, diet, or environment. Pets with this condition are often chronically, seriously debilitated, and many have concurrent disorders (e.g., parasites, infectious stomatitis). These animals are critically ill and require immediate and intensive hospitalization and treatment. The prognosis is guarded, as many of these pets have not eaten for several weeks. For animals with no history of diet, owner, or environmental change, and assuming the pet is eating an adequate diet and has a suitable environment, consider other etiologies (e.g., parasites, stomatitis, organ failure, obstruction).

Treatment

1. Incubation at 95–100 °F.
2. Fluids, orally and intracoelomically (15–25 mL/kg/day for maintenance [2]). Vomiting indicates a grave prognosis.
3. If no vomiting occurs, add 1 part electrolyte powder to 3 parts LRS (to slightly increase osmolality) and give orally at 15–25 mL/kg/day. Fluids are given intracoelomically prn (3).
4. If no vomiting occurs, switch the oral formula to Emeraid II or a similar product and give at 15–25 mL/kg/day. Start at a low dilution (1:6) and gradually increase to a dilution of 1:1 or 1:2 (3).
5. Offer fruits and vegetables once the iguana is able to tolerate the Emeraid at the stronger dilutions.
6. Treat other problems.

Fractures

Most fractures of the extremities, especially those caused by metabolic bone disease, are stable and heal rapidly as the disease resolves through treatment and improved diet (especially in the smaller iguanas; you may want to consider external stabilization with bandaging or tongue depressor splints in the larger iguanas) (1). Fractures of the vertebrae may or may not heal; often neurological impairment is permanent, but euthanasia should always be considered only as a last resort. Neurological impairment may respond to anti-inflammatory doses of corticosteroids. Give these pets time to assess the permanence of the neurological damage. Unstable limb fractures, as well as vertebral and mandibular fractures, can be immobilized. Femoral fractures (see Fig. 6.2) can be stabilized by binding the leg to the tail with Ethicon tape (7). The fractured rear leg is pulled straight back to lie alongside the tail; a tongue depressor can be placed on the opposite side of the tail to keep the tail from bending. Care should be taken not to occlude the cloaca (a hole can be cut in the tape to allow elimination if needed); petroleum jelly can be applied to the tape to keep it from soiling. Owners should keep the tape splint dry. The splint is removed in 4–6 weeks. Masking tape can be used for lizards less than 100 g.

Hypervitaminosis D

There exists some controversy on whether or not true "hypervitaminosis D" actually occurs in iguanas. Some research seems to indicate that reptiles are unable to absorb vitamin D from the intestinal tract. If this is true, then it is unlikely that iguanas would develop hypervitaminosis D from excess dietary vitamin D. Nevertheless, most current literature still discusses "hypervitaminosis D" when referring to the syndrome of severe hypercalcemia that seems to be related to an incorrect diet containing excess vitamin D. Therefore, this term is used in this text in the same fashion.

While hypovitaminosis D_3 often contributes to metabolic bone disease, hypervitaminosis D_3 is also harmful. This condition usually occurs when owners oversupplement with vitamins (only a light sprinkling is needed a few times a week) or give dog or cat food to their pets (both contain excessive amounts of vitamin D, as well as

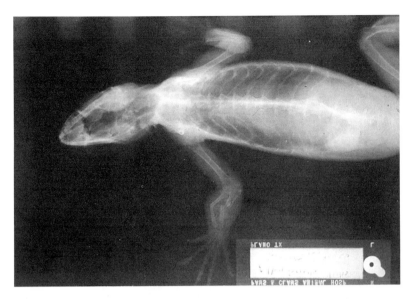

Fig. 6.2 *Folding fractures can be seen in metabolic bone disease.*

excess fat and protein). Periovulatory females can show marked hypercalcemia that has no significance.

Clinical signs are nonspecific and resemble many diseases; often, only anorexia and lethargy are seen. Radiographs occasionally reveal calcification of blood vessels or body organs. Blood tests for calcium usually reveal marked hypercalcemia (normal levels are 9–13 mg/dL) (3).

Treatment includes slowly correcting the diet, and hospitalization to correct the high calcium level. Fluids, steroids, and calcitonin are given to restore a normal blood calcium level. As with dogs and cats, treatment is often unsuccessful. Prevention is once again the best course.

Treatment (Empirical, Similar to Mammals with Vitamin D₃ Toxicosis)

1. Diuresis: Normally parenteral fluids are given in the amount of 15–25 mL/kg/day for maintenance (2). At minimum, this dose should be used to ensure hydration (using lactated Ringer's, or preferably physiologic, saline). Diuresis can be achieved by administering one to two times the maintenance amount.

2. Calcitonin: Two options can be considered:
   - Calcimar: Supplied as a stock solution of 200 IU/mL. It is diluted with sterile PSS to a final strength of 1.0 IU/mL and dosed at 3 units/2 kg SQ t.i.d.* (2).
   - Calcitonin (Calcimar, 50 IU/kg IM, two injections one week apart)** (5).

While it has not been reported in the literature as of this writing, treatment using furosemide for diuresis (5.0 mg/kg IV, IM s.i.d.–q.i.d. [2]) and corticosteroids (prednisolone 0.5–1.0 mg/kg s.i.d., avian dose [8]) to promote calcium excretion as in mammals may be helpful, especially if the combination of diuresis plus calcitonin fails to lower serum calcium levels appreciably.

Avascular Necrosis

Iguanas may be examined for avascular necrosis of the digits or tail. These necrotic areas appear darker than the surrounding tissue. Left untreated, the necrosis can spread cranially up the tail or digit.

The exact cause isn't always determined, but can include septicemia, mycotoxicosis, mycobacteriosis, a fungal infection, or retained skin after molting (1).

Treatment is simple when the condition is caught at an early stage, and involves amputation of the affected area. The tail can usually be fractured proximal to the avascular area by carefully breaking the tail through a fracture plane (which occurs *within* a vertebral body and not *between* vertebrae) after carefully incising the skin and musculature (see Fig. 6.3). The tail usually grows back if left unsutured.

---

*This regimen has been used by Frye and others, who noted a dramatic reduction of serum calcium. They recommended continuing treatment for several weeks to prevent rebound hypercalcemia. Monitoring of serum calcium levels is important to prevent hypocalcemia; diuresis is critical in the treatment of hypercalcemia.

**This dosage (50 IU/kg of either version of Calcimar) is used in metabolic bone disease as a parathyroid hormone antagonist. It has not been reported for use as a treatment of vitamin D_3 toxicity (hypercalcemia); it would be expected to be effective as it is substantially higher than Frye's dose. Mointoring of serum Calcium levels is important to prevent hypocalcemia.

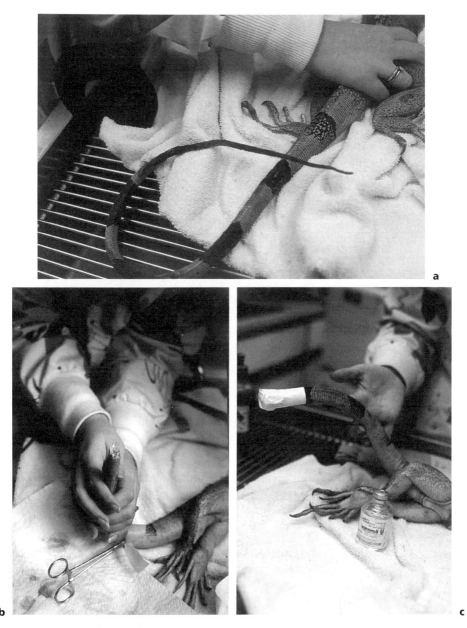

Fig. 6.3(a, b, & c) *Avascular necrosis of the tail is treated by amputating the tail. The tail is then bandaged (not sutured); the bandage can be removed in about 48 hours. If needed, owners can treat the tail topically with a spray bandage (such as Nexaband spray bandage) and an antibacterial ointment (Silvadene works well).*

Treatment

1. Amputation proximal to the necrotic area under general anesthesia or sedation and local anesthesia.
2. When possible, the tail should not be sutured as this procedure prevents regrowth (regenerated tails may be hyperpigmented). Toes should be sutured and are best amputated at the metacarpophalangeal or metatarsophalangeal junctions to ensure a cosmetic postoperative appearance (4). The tail is bandaged postoperatively for 1–2 days; Nexaband spray bandage can be used after the bandage has been removed for added protection.

■ **MISCELLANEOUS CONDITIONS**

Thiamine Deficiency (Hypovitaminosis B₁)

Iguanas that present with a flaccid paralysis of their limbs may have a thiamine deficiency. Other conditions to consider include dystocia in pregnant females and fractured vertebrae (typically secondary to metabolic bone disease). Clinical signs include flaccid paralysis, muscle tremors, anorexia, blindness, or sudden death. Thiamine deficiency can be caused by thiaminase in the diet (from fish or some plants) or prolonged antibiotic therapy or illness due to decreased intestinal synthesis (2).

Treatment

1. B-complex vitamins: 0.25–0.50 mL/kg IM to supply at least 25 mg/kg of thiamin (4). Used as needed (one injection may be all that is required).
2. Force feeding as needed with alfalfa pellets and/or *Lactobacillus* to reestablish intestinal microflora (2).

Cysts/Abscesses

Sebaceous inclusion cysts may be seen, especially in iguana tails. The cysts should be removed surgically. Diagnosis and treatment of an abscess involves lancing the abscess (often under anesthesia), flushing the cavity, and giving antibiotics (as based on culture and sensitivity tests). Cytological examination of cutaneous and subcutaneous nodules can be performed. Unlike mammalian abscesses, reptile abscesses contain firm caseated material rather than liquid pus (reptile heterophils lack the lysozymes to degrade and liquefy infectious materials). This structure may complicate the diagnosis of abscesses, although white blood cells and infectious organisms may be seen cytologically. Because the treatment (surgical removal) of the nodule is the same regardless of the cytological diagnosis, I rarely perform aspiration cytology on cutaneous or subcutaneous masses in reptiles unless the owner refuses surgical diagnosis and therapy. Antibiotic therapy could be attempted if surgery is refused based on a cytological diagnosis of an abscess, although this treatment is usually unsuccessful unless the abscess is opened and debrided.

Care should be taken as some abscesses are caused by zoonotic mycobacterial species.

Treatment

1. Debride the abscess under sedation or anesthesia. It may be possible to treat small abscesses under sedation and local anesthesia.
2. Flush the abscess cavity thoroughly with dilute povidone–iodine or chlorhexidine solution.
3. In contrast to the treatment of abscesses in dogs and cats, abscesses in reptiles are usually sutured (primary closure) due to the high incidence of infection of open wounds (contaminated wounds can, of course, be treated as open wounds). Darkening of the surrounding epidermis may be a possible consequence of healed surgical sites in reptiles.
4. A topical antibiotic ointment, such as Silvadene, can be used in the cavity until the abscess heals.
5. Strongly consider gram-staining and/or culturing abscesses. Anaerobic bacteria, fungi, and mycobacteria are often implicated as causes of abscesses.
6. On rare occasions, systemic antibiotics may be needed (see the discussion of treatment of infectious stomatitis) in cases of large or multiple abscesses. Antifungal therapy is used when needed.

Cystic Calculi

Cystic calculi occur when minerals from the diet form crystals that in turn form stones. These stones are typically composed of uric acid, which usually results from a diet that contains too much protein.

Blood in the droppings can be a sign of cystic calculi, as can abdominal swelling. Diagnosis is made by physical examination and radiography. Surgical removal of the stones is necessary, as is fluid therapy to prevent kidney damage; the animal's diet should be corrected to prevent reoccurrence of this condition. Often these iguanas are on diets that are too high in animal protein, such as dog or cat food. Switching them to a diet high in plant protein is essential.

Treatment

1. Cystotomy (similar to dogs and cats; avoid the central abdominal vein that runs on the ventral midline by making a paramedian incision).
2. Fluids prn (15–25 mL/kg/day for maintenance [2]).
3. Dietary correction.
4. Antibiotics if needed based on C&S.

Organ Failure

As with so many pets, renal and hepatic failure can be seen in iguanas; glomerulonephritis has also been reported. Iguanas with this condition are usually older pets; often the renal failure results from the same high protein diet that causes bladder stones. As with mammals, chronic renal and hepatic failure in iguanas is not reversible. With dogs and cats, we can often sustain life for a period of time. With exotic pets, the problem often isn't detected until it's too late.

Treatment, when attempted, involves aggressive fluid therapy and antibiotics. Lactulose and/or phosphate binders may be administered; the doses are extrapolated from mammalian doses. Intracoelomic lavage (dialysis) with 10–20 mL/kg of warm lactated Ringer's solution or "Reptile Ringer's" (see Appendix I) (removed in 5–30 minutes) may help in end-stage organ failure. Because the condition is often not detected until end-stage organ failure, prognosis is poor to grave.

Treatment

1. Fluids and force feeding.
2. Antibiotics (avoid nephrotoxic antibiotics).
3. Dietary correction.

Salmonella

While box turtles are infamous for this condition, any reptile can carry the *Salmonella* bacterium. Recently, reports have surfaced of *Salmonella* infections in iguana owners. This gram-negative bacterium can cause severe gastrointestinal disease or septicemia in reptiles and their owners. Most of the pet reptiles probably carry *Salmonella* as a part of their normal enteric flora, acting as asymptomatic carriers. True infection may occur when pets are stressed, resulting in an impaired immune system, which allows the normal flora to become pathogenic (2).

Salmonella infection can cause clinical disease in pet reptiles. Clinical signs include acute enteritis and septicemia, pneumonia, coelomitis, hypovolemic shock, and death (2). The feces of clinically ill reptiles may contain mucus and blood, and be colored a green–gray (2).

Prevention, through proper hygiene, is the best way to control the disease. Since most animals that carry the *Salmonella* bacterium aren't ill, they require no treatment (treating carriers often fails to eradicate the organism).

Dystocia

A common scenario in my practice involves female iguanas that become anorectic (or partially anorectic) during the breeding season (usually late fall and early winter) but are otherwise healthy. These animals have been found (on radiographs, microscopic fecal analysis, and blood tests) to be pre-ovulatory and without evidence of any disease. If the owners provide a suitable nesting environment, the iguanas will often lay the eggs. Most owners choose not to provide the nesting material so to avoid dealing with the eggs. No treatment has been necessary in these cases; the iguanas apparently resorb the yolks (fail to ovulate) and return to eating within a few months. Consultation with other veterinarians confirms my findings. Unless absolutely necessary, it is probably best to forgo force feeding these animals as this is stressful. The final decision on how to care for these animals rests with the veterinarian after assessing each individual case. I would recommend a complete workup to rule out other causes of anorexia before diagnosing this condition. If needed, an ovariohysterectomy can prevent the condition from recurring in those animals that are chronically affected.

Dystocia, or egg-binding, is occasionally encountered in iguanas. Unlike in mammals, dystocia in reptiles is often *not* a medical emergency; even with medical treatment, reptiles may not pass any retained eggs for a few days and still survive with no ill effects. However, iguanas with retained eggs quickly become depressed and immediate intervention is needed. Nevertheless, an examination or treatment should not be delayed, as early diagnosis and treatment improves the prognosis. Many owners don't detect early signs of dystocia (often the sex of the reptile isn't known even to the owner). The pet may not be examined until later in the course of the condition, when the problem may have become an emergency and require hospitalization and all the supportive care required by any "sick" reptile.

If the animal is known to be female, dystocia is more easily diagnosed. Often one or several eggs have already been passed, and the pet continues to strain as if trying to pass the remaining eggs. If no eggs have been passed, diagnosis is more difficult. Usually, the abdomen is obviously swollen. The owner may detect diarrhea, polyuria, or blood in the droppings. Definitive diagnosis requires radiographs; unless the shells are not calcified, the eggs are readily visible.

The cause of dystocia is often unknown, but poor diet, incorrect environmental temperature, improper nesting site, and internal disease are all contributing factors. For whatever reason, the uterus fails to expel the egg and it becomes stuck. Occasionally, the egg is too large to pass through the cloaca, resulting in dystocia.

Treatment is to relieve the dystocia and allow the iguana to pass the eggs. As with dogs and cats with dystocia, several treatment options are available.

Treatment

1. For eggs that are near the cloaca, lubrication of the cloaca and gentle manipulation can be tried first.
2. If lubrication and manipulation fail to correct the situation, calcium gluconate or lactate (10–50 mg/kg [4]) or calcium glycerophosphate and lactate (Calphosan, 1.0–2.5 mL/kg [100–250 mg/kg] [3]) and oxytocin (1–10 units [3,4]) IM are administered next. The iguana can be returned to the owner

with instructions to keep it quiet, avoid handling, and place it in a warm environment (85–90 °F). Most iguanas will pass eggs within 24–72 hours. Ovacentesis can be used prior to oxytocin and calcium, especially if the eggs appear enlarged (usually due to egg death and decomposition). Alternative therapies that reportedly have higher success rates use Calphosan (0.2–0.5 mL/kg IM, SQ) followed by arginine vasotocin (0.01–1.0 µm/kg IV, IP [20–50 mg/kg] [3]), or Inderal (1.0 µg/g) followed by vasotocin (500 ng/g [9]); arginine vasotocin is expensive, however, and not currently available except for research purposes.

3. If no eggs are passed after 24–72 hours, a repeat dose of calcium and oxytocin can be tried. Often, surgical removal is indicated at this point.

4. Ovariohysterectomy may be indicated. Some veterinarians recommend hysterectomy rather than ovariohysterectomy.

For an iguana that is obviously ill at the time of presentation, supportive care is needed. In addition, surgical intervention can be considered as a first option after the pet is stabilized.

The treatment of dystocia seems to evoke controversy among reptile practitioners. Many practitioners feel that oxytocin, especially if used as the sole agent, is unsuccessful in treating this condition. Oxytocin requires a hydrated uterine mucosa; prolonged egg retention results in a greater adherence of the uterine mucosa to the eggs as a result of mucosal dehydration. Some veterinarians feel that calcium is not useful prior to oxytocin injection but can be administered after several oxytocin injections. Multiple doses of oxytocin can result in uterine rupture if the etiology of the dystocia involves enlarged eggs. As with mammalian dystocia, treatment varies by practitioner and the treatment listed here is intended to serve as only a guideline.

Gastrointestinal Obstruction

Obstructions of the gastrointestinal tract can occur in iguanas. Obstructions can be caused by heavy parasite burdens (typically pinworms), foreign bodies (usually in young iguanas), cage bedding (especially if sand, shells, or corncob is used), or neoplasia. Symptoms are nonspecific but may include abdominal distention with tympany. Radiographs are needed to confirm obstructions and associated gaseous distention and ileus.

I have seen several cases of suspected "partial" obstruction in iguanas. These animals had a large amount of material in the stomach but no signs of intestinal ileus were present. The animals were anorectic and mildly lethargic upon presentation. Treatment with tap water enemas and gastric lavage with water and a small amount of vegetable oil, as well as SQ and intracoelomic fluid therapy, resolved the problem within a few days. One iguana had a secondary hepatopathy (increased SGOT) and also received antibiotics. Surgical intervention is often needed to correct the problem if a total obstruction is present.

Treatment

1. Supportive care prn.
2. Enemas and gastric lavage (force feeding) with tap water and a small amount of vegetable oil s.i.d.–b.i.d. may increase gastrointestinal motility and resolve the problem.
3. Exploratory laparotomy if the iguana is nonresponsive to supportive care or if a total obstruction is present.

Cloacal Prolapse

Cloacal prolapse can occur secondary to chronic straining, inflammation, infection, parasites, and dystocia. It may occur idiopathically. Repair is done under light sedation or isoflurane anesthesia. The prolapse can be replaced (often with a pursestring suture) or excised (via electrosurgery, which controls bleeding). Chronic prolapses require a cloacopexy.

Treatment

1. In mild cases, cleaning, lubrication, and replacement (similar to repair of avian cloacal prolapses with pursestring or transverse sutures if needed; I prefer the transverse closure) may work. Lidocaine gel, 50% dextrose, or glycerin may reduce the swelling. A linear cloacal incision (similar to an episiotomy) may reduce the prolapse. A fecal examination can rule out internal parasites.
2. Amputation (using electrosurgery to control bleeding if needed) is necessary if replacement is not feasible. The proce-

dure is not bloody and is fairly straightforward. Incise a small amount of tissue with a scalpel and suture that section before proceeding to the next section of tissue.

3. Cloacopexy becomes necessary in cases of chronic prolapse.

Hemipenile Prolapse

Prolapse of the hemipenes is occasionally encountered. Proposed etiologies include osteodystrophy; bacterial, parasitic, or fungal infections; trauma while breeding; and neurogenic defects of the penile or cloacal musculature. Differential diagnosis includes a prolapsed cloaca, intestine, and bladder. Treatment is similar to that for cloacal prolapse.

Treatment

1. In mild cases, cleaning, lubrication, and replacement (with pursestring suture if needed) may work. Preparation H, lidocaine gel, or 50% dextrose may reduce swelling.
2. Amputation (electrosurgically) is necessary if replacement is not feasible. The surgery is relatively straightforward, as the urethra empties into the cloaca and not the hemipenes (the hemipenes are used for reproduction only and not elimination of liquid waste).

Dysecdysis

Shedding problems are rarely seen in iguanas. Unlike snakes, iguanas usually shed in pieces rather than a single intact skin. Underlying causes (e.g., external parasites or dermatopathies), incorrect environment (e.g., humidity or temperature problems), and lack of substrates (needed for rubbing) should be corrected. Ecdysis is influenced both by environment (shedding frequency increases as temperature increases) and by endogenous hormones. Treatment involves soaking the pet to hydrate the retained skin and gently removing it.

Treatment

1. Soak the iguana in a shallow tub of water for 30–60 minutes (don't drown the iguana!). Use a wet towel to cover the iguana gently and act as an abrasive surface.

2. After soaking, place the pet in its cage with branches and rocks that can act as abrasive surfaces.
3. The skin can be gently peeled with forceps if necessary.

Rostral Abrasions

Occasionally, the rostrum (snout) of the iguana becomes abraded as the animal rubs its nose on the surface of its cage. This problem is created by the artificial environment associated with captivity. Often, providing a hiding place (box) will prevent the problem. Another solution involves a visual barrier of dark paint or plastic film applied to the lower (bottom) part of the glass front of the enclosure.

Treatment

1. Gentle cleansing (1% hydrogen peroxide, dilute chlorhexidine diacetate solution, or povidone–iodine solution).
2. Topical antibacterial medication.
3. Opsite spray bandage or Nexaband spray bandage can be used as a protective barrier.

Gout

In reptiles, uric acid is the end-product of protein metabolism and is excreted by the renal tubules. Hyperuricemia occurs when the kidneys are unable to filter uric acid from the blood; as a result, urates deposit in various body sites. Hyperuricemia can develop secondary to dehydration, high-protein diets, renal failure, and antibiotic (specifically aminoglycoside) usage (2,10). In one study in snakes, post-prandial uric acid levels peak (10–18 mg/dL) by the fourth day after feeding; levels returned to normal within 2 weeks after feeding (10). The same phenomenon may occur in other reptiles; uric acid levels should be evaluated in light of diet and time of recent feeding.

Visceral and articular gout may be seen in iguanas. Signs of this condition depend upon the site affected. Appendicular gout, which causes lameness and swelling, is less common than visceral gout (to which the liver, kidney, spleen, and pericardium are predisposed). Subcutaneous and sublingual uric acid deposits may also be seen in gout; obstipation can be seen if the intestines are involved. Joint aspirates may reveal uric acid crystals, confirming a diagnosis. Radiographs may reveal calcified tophi and/or joint swelling. Calcification of internal organs may be visible radiographically in visceral gout.

A common cause of this problem is a diet that contains excessive protein (often from dog or cat food or excessive amounts of animal-based protein). Dietary correction is needed; treatment is supportive. Allopurinol can be administered but reportedly has poor therapeutic success.

Treatment

1. Supportive (e.g., fluids).
2. Allopurinol.*
3. Avoidance of nephrotoxic drugs.
4. Dietary correction.

Burns

Burns are commonly seen as a result of the popular "Hot Rocks" and "Sizzle Stones." As discussed in chapter 3, these devices have no place in the reptile's environment. Most owners are surprised to learn that a reptile seeking warmth will lie on a hot surface and burn itself. Burns can also occur if the reptile is not protected from direct contact with a heat source such as a light bulb.

Treatment of burns is supportive and may include topical medication, parenteral antibiotics, and surgical debridement. Thermal burns tend to generate a large amount of scar tissue; healed skin may be depigmented (vitiligo). Healing skin may be retained during molting (dysecdysis).

Treatment

1. Local wound treatment involves water-soluble, antimicrobial wet dressings (dilute chlorhexidine diacetate solution, Dakin's solution) or ointments, including Betadine ointment, Furacin ointment, Sulfamylon ointment, or Silvadene cream (my preference). Opsite spray bandage or Nexaband spray bandage may be used to protect exposed tissue from desiccation and in-

---

* Allopurinol has proved ineffective in the few cases where it was used (2). A trial therapy may be indicated; an empirical dose (avian dose) uses one 100 mg tablet that is crushed in 10 mL of water; one drop of this mixture is given per 30 g of body weight q.i.d. (8). A dosage of 20 mg/kg PO s.i.d. for 2 weeks in turtles and snakes has been suggested; this regimen may be effective in iguanas (10).

fection. Particulate bedding material should not be employed because it adheres to wet dressings and ointments; clean cloth towels, paper towels, and butcher's paper are all acceptable.

2. Surgical debridement if needed.

3. Fluid therapy for extensive burns; as much as 75–150 mL/kg may be needed for the first 24–48 hours to ensure renal perfusion (2). Ascorbic acid (100–250 mg/kg s.i.d. [4]) and B-complex vitamins (0.25–0.50 mL/kg s.i.d. [4]) can be added to the fluids or given as individual injections.

4. Blood or plasma may be needed for extensive burns. Little information is available regarding blood component therapy in reptiles; extrapolation from canine, feline, or avian medicine is suggested.

5. Force feeding may be needed if the animal is anorectic; burns to the iguana's face may require an esophagostomy or gastrostomy tube for feeding.

6. Parenteral antibiotics are needed for all but the most minor, localized burns: (see Formulary for an in-depth discussion)

   • Amikacin: 2.5 mg/kg SQ, IM every 72 hours for 5–7 treatments* (2,4)
   • Piperacillin: 200–400 mg/kg IM q24 h* ** (4)
   • Cephalothin: 40–80 mg/kg dd b.i.d.* ** (2)
   • Trimethoprim–Sulfadiazine: 30 mg/kg SQ, IM q24 h for 10–14 treatments* (4)

You may want to use enrofloxacin (10 mg/kg IM q24h for 10–14 days) +/− amikacin as your initial antibiotic selection (4,6).

Regurgitation

Vomiting and regurgitation are rarely encountered medical problems in iguanas; these problems are not diseases themselves, but rather signs of serious underlying disease. When seen, a guarded to poor prognosis is warranted. Causes include improper environmental temperature, the anorexia/constipation/regurgitation syndrome, infectious disease, metabolic disease, intoxications, parasites, foreign

---

* Any of these agents is a rational choice for first-time antibiotic selection. Save Enrofloxacin for the more serious cases.   ** Combine with amikacin.

bodies, ulcerative disease, ingestion of putrified or contaminated (spoiled) food, abscesses, and neoplasia. Handling an iguana soon after eating may result in regurgitation.

A thorough diagnostic array of tests is often needed to determine the cause; a gastric lavage and microscopic examination are required in most cases. Treatment depends upon the cause of the problem.

Diarrhea

True diarrhea is rare in reptiles. What most owners call "diarrhea" is, in fact, polyuria. A fecal examination is always indicated in any pet with "diarrhea," as internal parasites are often the culprit in true diarrheic animals. Diet may also contribute to "diarrhea," particularly if large amounts of fruit are fed to the iguana. Bacteria, usually gram-negative pathogens, are also a possible cause of diarrhea in reptiles. Blood profiles, cytological examination and cultures of a colonic and/or gastric lavage, and radiographs may be necessary to determine a cause for the diarrhea. As is the case with vomiting, diarrhea is a clinical sign and not a disease.

■ REFERENCES

1. Boyer T. Common problems and treatment of green iguanas (*Iguana iguana*). Bull of ARAV, Premiere Issue: 8–11.
2. Frye F. Reptile care: An atlas of diseases and treatments, vols. I and II. Neptune City, NJ: TFH, 1991.
3. Anderson N. Husbandry and clinical evaluation of *Iguana iguana*. Compend Contin Educ Pract Vet, August 1991; 13:1265–1269.
4. Jenkins J. Medical management of reptile patients. Compend Contin Educ Pract Vet, June 1991; 13:980–988.
5. Mader D. Use of calcitonin in green iguanas, *Iguana iguana*, with metabolic bone disease. Bull of ARAV 3:5.
6. Boyer T. Common problems of box turtles (*Terrapene spp.*) in captivity. Bull of ARAV 2:9–16.
7. Stahl S. Fracture repair in iguanas. Bull of ARAV 5:4.
8. Ritchie B *et al.* Avian medicine: Principles and applications. Lake Worth: Wingers, 1994:458.
9. Suedmeyer WK. Noninfectious diseases of reptiles. Seminars in avian and exotic pet medicine, January 1995; 4:56–60.
10. Raiti P. Veterinary care of the common kingsnake, *Lampropeltis getula*. Bull of ARAV 5:11–18.

Diseases and Treatment of Snakes

▼ ▼ ▼ ▼ ▼ ▼ ▼ ▼

M OST OF the following information is applicable to all species of snakes. Because the ball python is the species of snakes most commonly seen in many practices, it was chosen as the representative species for the discussion.

■ COMMONLY SEEN CONDITIONS

Lumps and Bumps (1)

Owners often present a snake for diagnosis and treatment of a swelling in or on the body. Knowledge of normal anatomy is essential in preparing a differential diagnosis for intracoelomic swellings in snakes.

Anatomically, a snake's body can be divided into four quarters. A preliminary diagnosis can be made by knowing which quarter contains the swelling, and knowing which organs are contained within that quarter:

- First Quarter: Trachea, esophagus, heart (located at the junction of the first and second quarters).
- Second Quarter: Heart, liver, lung (right; the left lung is vestigial and occurs as an air sac in most snakes), stomach (located at the junction of the second and third quarters).
- Third Quarter: Stomach, gallbladder, gonads, small intestine, pancreas, spleen, adrenal glands.
- Fourth Quarter: Colon, kidneys, cloaca, cloacal opening (located at the junction of the fourth quarter and tail).
- Tail: Hemipenes (males), musk (scent, cloacal) glands (located at the junction of the fourth quarter and tail).

Confirmation often requires radiology, aspiration cytology, exploratory celiotomy, or a combination of these diagnostic techniques.

Conditions

Abscesses, tumors, and granulomas may occur in any quarter or anywhere on the snake's body.

In the first quarter, conditions may include cardiomyopathy, pericardial effusion, and pericarditis.

In the second quarter, problems may be attributable to recently ingested food, cryptosporidial hypertrophic gastritis (common), *Monocercomonas* gastritis, hepatitis, and intussusception.

Problems in the third quarter may include pancreatic and splenic abscesses and granulomas, *Monocercomonas* cholecystitis, and intussusception.

In the fourth quarter, lumps and bumps (see Fig. 7.1) may be caused by nephritis, renal gout (common), orchitis, obstipation/constipation (common), intussusception, eggs (common), fetal snakes,

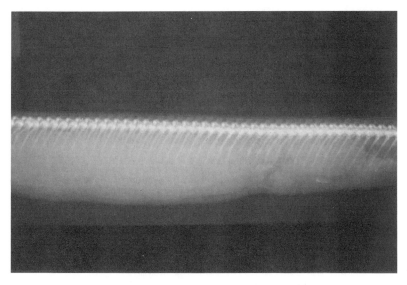

Fig. 7.1 *Soft tissue swelling seen radiographically in the fourth quarter of a snake. A renal abscess was diagnosed histopathologically.*

and cloacitis. Eggs occur in egg-laying species (pythons) and fetal snakes occur in live-bearing species (boas and garter snakes).

Treatment

Treatment depends upon the cause of the swelling. Many swellings will need to be treated surgically. Fecaliths, which are a common condition in snakes, can often be treated with enemas, especially if the swelling is just cranial to the cloaca. Soaking in warm water for a short period of time may stimulate defecation within 24 hours. The swelling is tentatively diagnosed as a fecalith when a red rubber feeding tube, introduced into the colon, does not easily pass into the colon. A lack of a recent bowel movement encourages suspicion of this problem. Tap water with or without a water-soluble lubricant or mild soap can be used to gently break down the fecalith (sedation may be needed) and allow its passage. The technique for an enema is similar to that used for a colonic wash.

Infectious Stomatitis

Infectious stomatitis, more commonly known as "mouth rot," is almost always caused by bacteria. While many species of bacteria are capable of causing the problem, *Pseudomonas* and *Aeromonas* are the most common culprits. Many veterinarians feel that this disease is always a secondary one, as *Pseudomonas* and *Aeromonas* are often normally present in a reptile's environment and body.

Although a filthy environment is a common cause of this problem, the cases I have seen have been from animals supposedly housed in clean environments. Other stressors that can cause infectious stomatitis include internal parasites, poor diet, improper environment and improper environmental temperature, shipping (as when a pet is brought into an owner's home after purchase), too little or too much handling, a too humid or too dry cage, and almost any other stress. The stress isn't always identified, but the pet should undergo a thorough diagnostic workup (treat the pet, not the disease!).

Early symptoms of disease that often go unnoticed by owners are petechial hemorrhages inside the oral cavity. These signs are often observed during a routine physical examination on an asymptomatic snake or in the oral cavity of a snake presented for another medical problem. Don't overlook these early lesions; begin treatment if they are detected. The later stages of disease reveal a large amount of frothy, bubbly mucus or a "cottage cheese" type of exudate. Many animals in the later stages are also anorectic and lethargic.

Diagnosis is fairly easy and is made by observation of the oral cavity. All obvious cases as well as suspected cases (when the character and amount of mucus seem slightly abnormal or petechial hemorrhages are seen) should be cultured. *Pseudomonas* and *Aeromonas* are often found in many normal reptiles, so their presence on a culture doesn't always mean the pet has, or will develop, mouth rot. Any heavy growth on a culture, particularly of a single pathogenic species of bacterium, should probably be treated.

Treatment varies with the severity of the disease. Snakes that are lethargic and anorectic need to be hospitalized. During hospitalization, these severely ill patients are given fluids, kept in an incubator (85–90 °F), and force-fed.

While awaiting the culture results, snakes are started on injectable antibiotics. The oral cavity is treated with a topical medication, such as dilute povidone–iodine solution, chlorhexidine diacetate solution, hydrogen peroxide, and/or Silvadene. Maxi-Guard gel, which has been used topically in iguanas, may be considered in snakes as well. Injectable atropine can be used if the mucus is thick and tenacious; many veterinarians feel that atropine helps to thin the mucus and allow for easier removal by the animal's body (2). Vitamin B complex injections are given. Vitamin C also seems clinically to help in many cases of infectious stomatitis (2).

The prognosis of infectious stomatitis depends upon several factors. If the animal is still eating and active, and no other diseases are detected, the prognosis is usually good. If signs are caught early, when only the petechial hemorrhages are seen, the prognosis is also very good. Animals that haven't eaten in several days or weeks, are weak and depressed, and have large amounts of mucus in their oral cavities are often septic and have a much poorer chance of recovery. Secondary problems, such as internal parasites, also need to be addressed. The environment should be corrected if necessary.

Treatment (Mild Cases)

1. Culture and sensitivity testing (possibly anaerobic as well as aerobic) of the oral cavity.
2. Begin antibiotic therapy with the following, pending C&S results: (see Formulary for an in-depth discussion).
   - Amikacin: 2.5 mg/kg SQ, IM every 72 hours for 5–7 treatments* (2,3)
   - Piperacillin: 200–400 mg/kg IM q24h* ** (3)
   - Cephalothin: 40–80 mg/kg dd b.i.d.* ** (2)
   - Trimethoprim–Sulfadiazine: 30 mg/kg SQ, IM q24h for 10–14 treatments* (3)
3. Oral therapy should include topical rinses performed as follows:
   - Dilute chlorhexidine solution (0.25–1.0%) (2)
   - Dilute povidone–iodine solution (1%) (2)
   - Acetic acid (vinegar) (dilute to a 0.5% solution) (2)
   - Hydrogen peroxide

   Rinses are given b.i.d.; the mouth is rinsed with plain water after the rinses are used. Alternating rinses (i.e., chlorhexidine solution day 1, peroxide day 2, acetic acid day 3, with the sequence repeated for the duration of treatment) may be helpful. You may decide to alternate rinses as follows: chlorhexidine in the morning, peroxide in the evening, and so on. Wear eye protection (goggles) and gloves, and have clients do the same when rinsing the oral cavity!
4. Topical Silvadene

Treatment (Severe Cases)

1. In addition to the treatment listed for mild cases, severely ill pets need hospitalization with fluid therapy (15–25 mL/kg/day for maintenance) (2), incubation (85–90 °F), and force feeding.
2. In addition, you may want to use enrofloxacin +/− amikacin as your initial antibiotic selection.
   - Enrofloxacin: 10 mg/kg IM q24h for 10–14 days (3,4)

---

* Any of these agents is a rational choice for first-time antibiotic selection. Save Enrofloxacin for the more serious cases.
** Combine with amikacin.

Many authors recommend parenteral fluids in any reptile receiving aminoglycosides, and to a lesser extent piperacillin and cephalosporins, to prevent renal damage (2).

Anorexia

Snakes may refuse to feed for a variety of reasons. For example, newly acquired pythons may refuse to feed. Frequent handling, especially of recently purchased snakes, is very stressful and can cause anorexia. Failure to provide a hide box, a heat source, and possibly UV lighting may also cause anorexia; a proper thermal gradient must exist in the cage, and water must be available 24 hours a day. In addition, snakes that are shedding or pregnant won't eat, and some species of snakes (both males and females) will refuse to feed during the breeding season ("breeding season anorexia" is common in some species of male snakes of the *Boa* and *Python* genera [23]). Sick snakes won't eat. The proper diet must be offered before a snake will feed (e.g., some ball pythons won't eat mice or rats and need to be fed gerbils, which are their natural prey in the wild).

The only way to determine whether or not anorexia in a snake is "normal" (temporary, physiologic) or "abnormal" (pathologic, a sign of serious underlying disease), is through the use of laboratory tests. In general, I recommend a complete physical examination (paying careful attention to the history given by the owner), a microscopic fecal examination (on a sample collected by a colonic wash), and a complete blood count and biochemical profile.

If a specific disease is detected, it may be amendable to treatment. Otherwise, if no etiology for the anorexia is discovered, the owner can try various feeding regimens (see the section on feeding snakes in chapter 4). Alternatively, the snake can be force fed (see pg 35) or given an appetite stimulating dose of metronidazole via stomach tube (50–125 mg/snake). (2).

Respiratory Disease

Respiratory diseases are often secondary to some other condition, such as lungworms or infectious stomatitis. Respiratory disease can be anything as mild as rhinitis or as severe as pneumonia; causative organisms include bacteria (most commonly), fungi, viruses, or parasites. Lack of a diaphragm prevents active coughing from the air-sac-like lungs of reptiles. The mainstem bronchi and trachea enter the lungs more cranially than in mammals. These factors favor the retention of respiratory secretions in the lower airways, which means that simple respiratory infections are more prone to developing into pneumonia in reptiles than in mammals. Conversely, muscular anaerobiasis (glycolic respiration) is remarkable in reptiles; they can often survive respiratory infections that would prove fatal to animals lacking anaerobic respiratory capabilities.

Many "simple" respiratory infections in reptiles are actually signs of serious lower respiratory disease and may require aggressive treatment. While the prognosis for such infections is always guarded, many reptiles will survive *if* appropriate aggressive treatment is instituted. Any reptile that is anorectic and lethargic and has respiratory signs (e.g., sneezing, wheezing, mucopurulent nasal discharge, dyspnea, open-mouth breathing) should be assumed to have pneumonia until proved otherwise and treated aggressively. Many of these pets are gravely ill and hospitalization is essential. Hospitalized snakes are kept in an incubator and given fluids and force feeding. Cultures of the respiratory tract are taken, and a tracheal and colonic wash are performed to examine for parasites. Injectable antibiotics are administered. Once the snake begins to improve, the owner can continue antibiotic injections at home.

Treatment

1. Maintain hydration with intracoelomic fluids at 15–25 mL/kg/day for maintenance (2).
2. Force-feed as needed.
3. Begin antibiotic therapy with the following, pending C&S results: (see Formulary for an in-depth discussion).
   - Amikacin: 2.5 mg/kg SQ, IM every 72 hours for 5–7 treatments* (2,3)
   - Piperacillin: 200–400 mg/kg IM q24h* ** (3)
   - Cephalothin: 40–80 mg/kg dd b.i.d.* ** (2)

* Any of these agents is a rational choice for first-time antibiotic selection. Save enrofloxacin for the more serious cases.
** Combine with amikacin.

- Trimethoprim–Sulfadiazine: 30 mg/kg SQ, IM q24h for 10–14 treatments* (3)

You may want to use enrofloxacin (10 mg/kg IM q24h for 10–14 days) +/− amikacin as your initial antibiotic selection (3,4).

4. Perform a tracheal wash, cytology, and culture and sensitivity test as needed.
5. Perform a fecal flotation.
6. Maintain a warm (85–90 °F) environment.
7. Nebulization using Amikacin or Gentamicin may be indicated. Regimens follow those used in birds and mammals. Some veterinarians advocate adding a bronchodilator, cromalyn sodium, and/or acetylcysteine to the nebulizing solution.
8. Oxygen therapy as needed.
9. Furosemide (5 mg/kg IV, IM prn [2]) can reduce respiratory fluids; parenteral fluids should be used concurrently with diuretics.
10. Atropine (0.04 mg/kg PO, IV, IM, SQ prn [2]) can dry mucous membranes.

Septicemia

Septicemia can result as a direct infection of the blood or after a localized infection (infectious stomatitis, for example) spreads hematogenously. Septic animals are gravely ill and require hospitalization and intensive therapy.

Septic snakes are lethargic and refuse to feed. They may exhibit reduced muscle tone or contractions when handled during the examination. Often these animals have pinpoint hemorrhagic areas on their mucus membranes and ventral scales (see Fig. 7.2).

Supportive care is similar to that provided to snakes hospitalized for respiratory infections.

Treatment

1. Maintain hydration with intracoelomic fluids at 15–25 mL/kg/day (2).
2. Force-feed as necessary.

---

* Any of these agents is a rational choice for first-time antibiotic selection. Save enrofloxacin for the more serious cases.

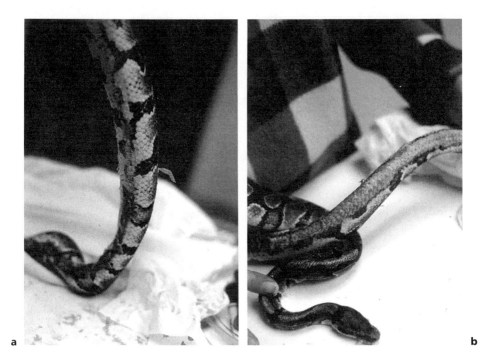

a   b

Fig. 7.2(a & b) *Erosion of the ventral scales revealing underlying tissue is seen in the photographs of a ball python with septicemia.*

3. Begin antibiotic therapy with the following, pending C&S results: (see Formulary for an in-depth discussion).
   - Amikacin: 2.5 mg/kg SQ, IM every 72 hours for 5–7 treatments* (2,3)
   - Piperacillin: 200–400 mg/kg IM q24h* ** (3)
   - Cephalothin: 40–80 mg/kg dd b.i.d.* ** (2)
   - Trimethoprim–Sulfadiazine: 30 mg/kg SQ, IM q24h for 10–14 treatments* (3)

   You may want to use enrofloxacin (10 mg/kg IM q24h for 10–14 days) +/− amikacin as your initial antibiotic selection (3,4).

4. Perform a tracheal wash, cytology, and culture and sensitivity test as needed.

5. Perform a fecal flotation after collection with a colonic wash.

6. Maintain a warm (85–90 °F) environment.

* Any of these agents is a rational choice for first-time antibiotic selection. Save enrofloxacin for the more serious cases.
** Combine with amikacin.

Dysecdysis

Snakes normally shed their entire skin in one piece. While the timing varies, most snakes shed every 1–2 months. Snakes that seem to shed constantly are often found to have hyperthyroidism. Younger animals shed more frequently than older ones. Shedding is dependent upon many factors, including proper feeding and environment and the absence of disease. As noted earlier, shedding is stressful to snakes and most will not eat during the shedding process.

Shedding generally takes place through the following process: One to two weeks before shedding, the snake may become inactive and its eyes turn a cloudy blue or gray color. The skin takes on a dull appearance. The eyes stay blue for about a week, and then become clear again; shedding begins within 2–7 days after this change. The skin covering the head is shed first, and then the snake rolls out of its old skin. After shedding, the snake is usually very hungry and thirsty. Because shedding is stressful, the snake should not be handled during this period unless an emergency occurs or medical treatment becomes necessary.

Dysecdysis—difficult shedding—occurs when the snake fails to shed all or part of its skin. If part of the skin fails to shed, treatment is usually simple and straightforward. Placing the snake in a container (such as a Styrofoam or plastic cooler) with wet towels for a few hours normally hydrates the skin; the towel acts as a mild abrasive surface and the crawling snake is able to complete shedding. Occasionally, you may have to use a moist towel to gently rub off the old skin.

On rare occasions, the eye caps (spectacles) will remain after a shed. Care should be exercised when removing retained spectacles, as the cornea can be severely damaged if the spectacles are pulled off in a haphazard manner.

Excess shedding (molting) has been reported in some snakes. These animals remain in a constant "shed mode" or have an extremely short (1- to 2-week) intershed interval. The most common cause of molting is reported to be hyperthyroidism. Treatment is with methimazole (1.0–1.25 mg/kg PO s.i.d. for 30 days [2]) or propylthiouracil (10 mg/kg PO s.i.d. for 21–30 days [2]). Thyroid values should be determined before and during treatment to allow dosage adjustment. An effort should be made to decrease the dosage gradually after roughly 4 months of treatment. If excess shedding resumes, continuous therapy at the lowest maintenance dosage possibly may be needed.

Prior to shedding, some boas and pythons are brought to veterinarians because of wheezing, mild cephalic edema, ventral erythema, and suspected respiratory disease. If no other signs of respiratory disease (clogged nares, open-mouth breathing, chronic anorexia, infectious stomatitis) are seen, these snakes do not require treatment but should be reexamined after shedding is completed. In most cases, the signs will have lessened or resolved (5).

Treatment

1. Soak the snake in a shallow tub of water for 30–60 minutes; a small amount of mild dishwashing soap or DSS can act as a surfactant and increase the wetability of the old skin. A wet towel can be used to gently cover the snake (or two towels can "sandwich" the snake) and to act as an abrasive surface.
2. After soaking, place the snake in its cage with branches and rocks available to act as abrasive surfaces.
3. The skin can be gently peeled with forceps if needed.
4. To remove retained spectacles, either the entire snake can be soaked or warm, moist cotton packs can be applied to the eyes for 10–15 minutes (some veterinarians like to generously soak the spectacles with contact lens solution). The edge of the retained spectacle is gently grasped and lifted with iris forceps or a hemostat. Mild force is usually all that is needed; excessive force can permanently damage the corneas.

Prey Attacks

Many owners are astonished to discover that a prey item such as a mouse or rat will attack a snake! Unfortunately, such events happen with some frequency. Many of these wounds are serious, and some may even prove fatal. The situation can be prevented by offering snakes only stunned or killed prey, or by carefully watching the snake for several minutes after the live prey is put into the cage. Prey that isn't eaten within 10–15 minutes should be removed immediately and offered at a later time.

Because most snakes are sight and olfactory feeders, loss of the tongue can be devastating; hand feeding may be required for life (2). Snakes will usually manage well without sight in the event that both eyes are lost due to the attack (2). Rodent bites heal slowly and lead to scar formation and wound contraction at the skin edges; skin sutures are best removed as soon as the risk of dehiscence no longer exists to lessen dermal contraction (2). Mycotic infections are also a danger with rodent bites. Wounds that are not healing should be examined cytologically and cultured for fungi; ketoconazole may be indicated.

Treatment

1. Suturing is undertaken if possible; skin grafting may also be needed. Some wounds can be managed only as open wounds.
2. Flush with dilute chlorhexidine diacetate solution or povidone–iodine daily solution.
3. Topical antibiotics, such as Silvadene cream.
4. Systemic antibacterial therapy, pending C&S results: (see Formulary for an in-depth discussion).
   - Amikacin: 2.5 mg/kg SQ, IM every 72 hours for 5–7 treatments* (2,3)
   - Piperacillin: 200–400 mg/kg IM q24h* ** (3)
   - Cephalothin: 40–80 mg/kg dd b.i.d.* ** (2)
   - Trimethoprim–Sulfadiazine: 30 mg/kg SQ, IM q24h for 10–14 treatments* (3)

   You may want to use enrofloxacin (10 mg/kg IM q24h for 10–14 days) +/− amikacin as your initial antibiotic selection (3,4).
5. Apply topical spray bandages such as Opsite or Nexaband for protection; repeat prn.
6. With massive loss of soft tissue or bone, lesions should be covered with wet dressings. The most practical method is to place the snake in a Styrofoam container and cover the pet with clean towels soaked in dilute chlorhexidine diacetate for

---

* Any of these agents is a rational choice for first-time antibiotic selection. Save enrofloxacin for the more serious cases.
** Combine with amikacin.

several days. Condoms can be used as a bandage for snakes (2).

7. Bedding should be changed to paper towels, butcher paper, or soft cloth towels; remove branches and other rough surfaces.

8. Traumatic lesions to the tongue can usually be treated conservatively with topical petrolatum-based ophthalmic ointment containing antibiotics and corticosteroids placed into the space between the sheath and lingual surfaces. Excess scarring that develops despite topical therapy can be treated with small amounts of methylprednisolone acetate or triamcinolone acetonide injected intralesionally with a 27–30 gauge needle. If the tongue cannot be retracted into the sheath, surgical therapy is indicated (2).

■ LESS COMMON CONDITIONS

External/Internal Parasites

See chapter 9, "Parasites," for a complete discussion of this problem.

Organ Failure

As with so many pets, renal and hepatic failure can be seen in snakes. The snakes so affected are usually older pets. Gout or treatment with aminoglycoside antibiotics can cause organ failure. As with mammals, chronic renal and hepatic failure is not reversible. With dogs and cats, we can often sustain life for a period of time. With exotic pets, the problem often isn't detected until it's too late. Treatment, when attempted, involves aggressive fluid therapy and antibiotics. Lactulose and phosphate binders (with dosage extrapolated from avian doses) may be tried. Because this condition is often detected only as end-stage organ failure, prognosis is poor to grave.

Treatment

1. Fluids (15–25 mL/kg/day for maintenance [2]) and force feeding.

2. Antibiotics may be needed in acute episodes or if organ failure is associated with an infection (avoid nephrotoxic antibiotics).

3. Dietary correction.

Salmonella

While box turtles are infamous for this condition, any reptile can carry the *Salmonella* bacterium. This gram-negative bacterium can cause severe gastrointestinal disease or septicemia in both reptiles and their owners. Most pet reptiles probably carry *Salmonella* as a part of their normal enteric flora, acting as asymptomatic carriers. True infection may occur when pets are stressed, resulting in an impaired immune system that allows the normal flora to become pathogenic (2). *Salmonella* infection can cause clinical disease in pet reptiles. Clinical signs include acute enteritis and septicemia, pneumonia, coelomitis, hypovolemic shock, and death (2). The feces of clinically ill reptiles may contain mucus and blood, and be colored green–gray (2).

Prevention, through proper hygiene, is the best way to control this disease. Because most animals that carry the bacterium aren't ill, they require no treatment (treating carriers often fails to eradicate the organism).

Dystocia

Dystocia, or egg-binding, is occasionally encountered in snakes. Unlike in mammals, dystocia is often *not* a medical emergency in reptiles; even with medical treatment, reptiles may not pass any retained eggs for a few days and still survive with no ill effects. An examination or treatment should not be delayed, however, as early diagnosis and treatment improves the prognosis. Many owners don't detect early signs of dystocia (often the sex of the reptile isn't known even to the owner). As a result, the pet may not be examined until later in the course of the condition, when the problem may be an emergency requiring hospitalization and all of the supportive care required by any "sick" reptile.

If the animal is known to be female, dystocia is more easily diagnosed. Often one or several eggs have already been passed, and the pet continues to strain as if trying to pass the remaining eggs. If no eggs have been passed, diagnosis is more difficult. Usually, the abdomen is obviously swollen. The owner may notice polyuria, diarrhea, or blood in the droppings. Definitive diagnosis requires radiographs; eggshells are poorly calcified when compared with chelonian eggs.

The cause of dystocia is often unknown. Poor diet, incorrect environmental temperature, lack of exercise (and, therefore, of muscle tone), lack of a secluded area in which to lay eggs, and internal disease are all contributing factors, however. For some reason, the uterus fails to expel the egg, which becomes stuck. Occasionally, the egg is too big to pass through the cloaca and results in dystocia.

Not all snakes lay eggs. Pythons are oviparous and lay eggs; boas, being viviparous species, bear live young. Treatment is to relieve the dystocia and allow the snake to pass the eggs.

Treatment

1. For eggs that are near the cloaca, lubrication of the cloaca and gentle manipulation can be tried first.
2. If lubrication and manipulation fail to correct the situation, calcium gluconate or lactate (10–50 mg/kg [3]) or calcium glycerophosphate and lactate (Calphosan, 1.0–2.5 mL/kg [100–200 mg/kg] [3]) and oxytocin (1–10 units, or 5 units/kg [3,6]) IM are tried next. The snake can be returned to the owner with instructions to keep it quiet, avoid handling, and place the snake in a warm environment (85 °F). Most snakes will pass eggs within 24–72 hours. Ovacentesis can be used prior to oxytocin and calcium, especially if the eggs appear enlarged (usually due to egg death and decomposition). Dehydrated patients should be rehydrated prior to the use of ecbolic agents.
3. If no eggs are passed after 24–72 hours, a repeat dose of calcium and oxytocin can be tried. Often, surgical removal is indicated at this point.
4. Alternatively, Calphosan (0.2–0.5 mL/kg IM or SQ [20–50 mg/kg]) followed by arginine vasotocin (0.01–1.0 µm/kg IV or IP) can be used (6). Inderal (1.0 µg/g) followed by vasotocin [7] (500 ng/g) has also reportedly been used. The literature has suggested greater efficacy with this protocol than with calcium and oxytocin; arginine vasotocin is expensive, however, and is not currently available except for research.

5. If these steps fail, ovariohysterectomy may be indicated. Some authors recommend hysterectomy rather than ovario-hysterectomy.

For snakes that are obviously ill at the time of presentation, supportive care is needed. In addition, surgical intervention can be considered as a first option after the pet is stabilized.

The treatment of dystocia seems to evoke controversy among reptile practitioners. Many veterinarians feel that oxytocin, especially if used as the sole agent, is unsuccessful in treating dystocia in snakes (2). Oxytocin requires a hydrated uterine mucosa; prolonged egg retention results in a greater adherence of the uterine mucosa to the eggs as a result of mucosal dehydration. Some practitioners believe that calcium is not useful prior to oxytocin injection but can be tried after several oxytocin injections. Multiple doses of oxytocin can result in uterine rupture if the etiology of the dystocia is enlarged eggs. As with mammalian dystocia, treatment varies by practitioner and the treatment listed here is intended to serve as only a guideline.

Gastrointestinal Obstruction

Obstructions of the gastrointestinal tract can occur in snakes because of the presence of parasites (typically *Cryptosporidium* gastric granulomas), foreign bodies, cage bedding (especially if sand, shells, or corncob is used), neoplasia, or, most commonly, fecaliths. Symptoms may include regurgitation, anorexia, lethargy, or swelling somewhere along the length of the snake (see the earlier section, "Lumps and Bumps"). Radiographs can be helpful in diagnosis; if the obstruction is just cranial to the cloaca and is presumed to be a fecalith, radiographs may not be needed. Surgical intervention may be needed to correct the problem, as no effective treatment for cryptosporidiosis exists at this time.

Treatment

1. Supportive care prn.
2. Exploratory laparotomy.
3. Enema (fecaliths).

Cloacal Prolapse

Cloacal prolapse can occur secondary to chronic straining, inflammation, infection, parasites, and dystocia. On rare occasions, it may occur idiopathically. Repair is done under light sedation or isoflurane anesthesia. The prolapse can be replaced (often with a pursestring or transverse suture) or excised (with electrosurgery being used to control bleeding). Chronic prolapses require a cloacopexy.

Treatment

1. In mild cases, cleaning, lubrication, and replacement (with pursestring suture if needed) may work. Lidocaine gel, 50% dextrose, or glycerin may reduce the swelling. A linear cloacal incision may be needed to reduce the swelling; the incision is sutured after cloacal replacement. A fecal examination can rule out internal parasites.
2. Amputation (using electrosurgery as needed) or cloacopexy is needed in chronic cases; necrotic tissue should be amputated. The procedure is not bloody and is fairly straightforward. Incise a small amount of tissue with a scalpel and suture that section before proceeding to the next section of tissue.

Hemipenile Prolapse

Prolapse of the hemipenes is occasionally encountered in snakes. Proposed etiologies include osteodystrophy; bacterial, parasitic, or fungal infections; trauma while breeding; and neurogenic defects of the penile or cloacal musculature. Treatment is similar to that of cloacal prolapse. Differential diagnosis includes prolapsed cloaca, intestine, and bladder.

1. In mild cases, cleaning, lubrication, and replacement (with pursestring suture if needed) may work. Preparation H, lidocaine gel, or 50% dextrose may reduce swelling (6).
2. Amputation (electrosurgically) is advised if replacement is not feasible.

Rostral Abrasions

Occasionally, the rostrum (snout) of the snake becomes abraded as the animal rubs its nose on the surface of its cage. This problem is created by the artificial environment associated with captivity. Often, a hiding place (box) will prevent this condition. Another solution involves a visual barrier of dark paint or plastic film applied to the lower (bottom) part of the glass front of the enclosure.

Treatment

1. Gentle cleansing of the abrasion with hydrogen peroxide, dilute chlorhexidine diacetate, or povidone–iodine solution.
2. Topical antibacterial medication.
3. Opsite spray bandage or Nexaband spray bandage can be used as a wound dressing.

Gout

In reptiles, uric acid is the end-product of protein metabolism and is excreted by the renal tubules. Hyperuricemia occurs when the kidneys are unable to filter uric acid from the blood; as a result, urates deposit in various body sites. Hyperuricemia can develop secondary to dehydration, high-protein diets, renal failure, and antibiotic (specifically, aminoglycoside) usage (2,8). In one study in snakes, post-prandial uric acid levels peaked (10–18 mg/dL) by the fourth day after feeding; levels returned to normal within 2 weeks after feeding (8). The same phenomenon may occur in other reptiles; uric acid levels should be evaluated in light of diet and time of recent feeding.

Visceral and articular gout may be seen in snakes, with signs depending upon the site affected. Appendicular gout, which causes lameness and swelling, is less common than visceral gout (to which the liver, kidney, spleen, and pericardium are predisposed). Subcutaneous and sublingual uric acid deposits may also be seen in gout; obstipation can be seen if the intestines are involved. Joint aspirates may reveal uric acid crystals, confirming a diagnosis. Radiographs may reveal calcified tophi and/or joint swelling. Calcification of internal organs may be visible radiographically in visceral gout. A common cause is an incorrect diet (often consisting of dog or cat food or excessive amounts of animal-based protein). Dietary correction is needed; treatment is supportive. Allopurinol can be tried but reportedly has poor success (2).

Treatment

1. Supportive (e.g., fluids).
2. Allopurinol.*
3. Avoid nephrotoxic drugs.

Burns

Burns are commonly seen in snakes as a result of the popular "Hot Rocks" or "Sizzle Stones." As noted earlier, these devices have no place in the reptile's environment. Most owners are surprised to learn that a reptile seeking warmth will lay on a hot surface and burn itself. Burns can also occur if the reptile is not protected from direct contact with a heat source such as a light bulb. Treatment is supportive and may include topical medication, parenteral antibiotics, and surgical debridement. Thermal burns tend to form large amounts of scar tissue; healed skin may be depigmented (vitiligo). Healing skin may be retained during molting (dysecdysis).

Treatment

1. Local wound treatment involves water-soluble, antimicrobial wet dressings (dilute chlorhexidine diacetate solution, Dakin's solution) or ointments, including Betadine ointment, Furacin ointment, Sulfamylon ointment, or Silvadene cream (my preference). Opsite spray bandage or Nexaband spray bandage may be used to protect exposed tissue from desiccation and infection. Particulate bedding material should not be used because it adheres to wet dressings and ointments; clean cloth towels, paper towels, and butcher's paper are acceptable materials.

---

*Allopurinol was ineffective in the few cases where it was used for reptile gout. A trial therapy may be indicated; an empirical avian dose uses one 100 mg tablet that is crushed in 10 mL of water; one drop of this mixture is given per 30 g of body weight q.i.d. (8). A dosage of 20 mg/kg PO s.i.d. for 2 weeks in turtles and snakes has been suggested; this regimen may also be effective in iguanas (9).

2. Surgical debridement if needed.

3. Fluid therapy for extensive burns; as much as 75–150 mL/kg may be needed for the first 24–48 hours to ensure renal perfusion. Ascorbic acid and B-complex vitamins can be added to the fluid (2).

4. Blood or plasma may be required for extensive burns. Little information is available regarding blood component therapy in reptiles; extrapolation from canine, feline, and avian medicine is suggested.

5. Parenteral antibiotics are needed for all but the most minor, localized burns: (see Formulary for an in-depth discussion).
   - Amikacin: 2.5 mg/kg SQ, IM every 72 hours for 5–7 treatments* (2,3)
   - Piperacillin: 200–400 mg/kg IM q24h* ** (3)
   - Cephalothin: 40–80 mg/kg dd b.i.d.* ** (2)
   - Trimethoprim–Sulfadiazine: 30 mg/kg SQ, IM q24h for 10–14 treatments* (3)

   You may want to use enrofloxacin (10 mg/kg IM q24h for 10–14 days) +/− amikacin as your initial antibiotic selection (3,4).

Necrotizing Dermatitis (Blister Disease)

This condition is usually seen in snakes kept in humid or wet environments. The moisture promotes the overgrowth of pathogens (typically *Aeromonas* and *Pseudomonas*, but occasionally fungi) that are responsible for the infection. Fluid-filled vesicles develop in the epidermis and may progress to visible caseation necrosis and subcutaneous abscessation. Left untreated, snakes become septic and die.

Treatment

1. Culture and sensitivity test of vesicular fluid.

2. Gentle washes/soaks with chlorhexidine diacetate scrub or povidone–iodine scrub (diluted to one-fourth strength).

---

* Any of these agents is a rational choice for first-time antibiotic selection. Save enrofloxacin for the more serious cases.
** Combine with amikacin.

3. Daily diluted chlorhexidine diacetate soaks (0.5–1.0%).
4. Begin antibiotic therapy with the following, pending C&S results: (see Formulary for an in-depth discussion).
    *   Amikacin: 2.5 mg/kg SQ, IM every 72 hours for 5–7 treatments* (2,3)
    *   Piperacillin: 200–400 mg/kg IM q24h* ** (3)
    *   Cephalothin: 40–80 mg/kg dd b.i.d.* ** (2)
    *   Trimethoprim–Sulfadiazine: 30 mg/kg SQ, IM q24h for 10–14 treatments* (3)

    You may want to use enrofloxacin (10 mg/kg IM q24h for 10–14 days) +/− amikacin as your initial antibiotic selection (3,4).
5. Disinfect the snake's environment.
6. Supportive care (e.g., fluids, force feeding, incubation).

Regurgitation

Vomiting or regurgitation is a medical problem that is rarely encountered in reptiles. When seen, it warrants a guarded to poor prognosis. Causes include improper environmental temperature, infectious disease, metabolic disease, intoxications, parasites (especially *Cryptosporidium*), foreign bodies, ulcerative disease, ingestion of putrified or contaminated (spoiled) food, abscesses, and neoplasia (4). Handling a snake soon after eating (within 24–72 hours) often results in regurgitation (2). A thorough battery of diagnostic tests is often needed to determine the cause of this problem; a gastric lavage and microscopic examination is critical in many cases. (Radiography, when indicated, should be performed prior to gastric lavage.) Treatment depends upon the cause. Vomiting and regurgitation are not diseases themselves, but signs of disease!

Diarrhea

Diarrhea is rare in reptiles. A fecal examination is always indicated in any pet with diarrhea, as often internal parasites are the culprits. Bacteria, usually gram-negative pathogens, are also a possible cause

---

* Any of these agents is a rational choice for first-time antibiotic selection. Save enrofloxacin for the more serious cases.
** Combine with amikacin.

of diarrhea in reptiles. In addition, cryptosporidiosis and (occult) coccidiosis are possibilities. A prophylactic trial of a coccidiostat may be indicated. Blood profiles, cytological examination and cultures of a colonic and/or gastric lavage, and radiographs may be necessary to determine a cause for the diarrhea. Diarrhea, like regurgitation, is a clinical sign rather than a disease.

Abscesses

Diagnosis and treatment of an abscess involves lancing the abscess (often under anesthesia), flushing the cavity, and giving antibiotics (as based on culture and sensitivity tests). Cytological examination of cutaneous and subcutaneous nodules can be performed. Unlike mammalian abscesses, reptile abscesses contain firm caseated material rather than liquid pus (reptile heterophils lack the lysozymes to degrade and liquefy infectious materials). This structure may complicate the diagnosis of abscesses, although white blood cells and infectious organisms may be seen cytologically. Because the treatment (surgical removal) of the nodule is the same regardless of the cytological diagnosis, I rarely perform aspiration cytology on cutaneous or subcutaneous masses in reptiles unless the owner refuses surgical diagnosis and therapy. Antibiotic therapy could be tried if surgery is refused based on a cytological diagnosis of an abscess, although this treatment is usually unrewarding unless the abscess is opened and debrided.

Care should be taken as some abscesses are caused by zoonotic mycobacterial species.

Treatment

1. Debride the abscess under sedation or anesthesia. It may be possible to treat small abscesses under sedation and local anesthesia.
2. Flush the abscess cavity thoroughly with dilute povidone–iodine or chlorhexidine diacetate solution.
3. In contrast to the treatment of abscesses in dogs and cats, abscesses in reptiles are usually sutured (primary closure) due to the high incidence of infection of open wounds (contaminated wounds can, of course, be treated as open wounds).

Darkening of the surrounding epidermis may be a possible consequence of healed surgical sites in reptiles.

4. A topical antibiotic ointment, such as Silvadene, can be used in the cavity until the abscess heals.

5. Strongly consider gram-staining and/or culturing abscesses. Anaerobic bacteria, fungi, and mycobacteria are often implicated as causes of abscesses.

6. On rare occasions, systemic antibiotics may be needed (see the discussion of infectious stomatitis) in cases of large or multiple abscesses. Antifungal therapy is used when necessary.

■ **REFERENCES**

1. Russo E. Diagnosis and treatment of lumps and bumps in snakes. Compend Contin Educ Pract Vet, August 1987; 9:795–802.

2. Frye F. Reptile care: An atlas of diseases and treatments, vols. I and II. Neptune City, NJ: TFH, 1991.

3. Jenkins J. Medical management of reptile patients. Compend Contin Educ Pract Vet, June 1991; 13:980–988.

4. Boyer T. Common problems of box turtles (*Terrapene spp.*) in captivity. Bull of ARAV 2:9–16.

5. Boyer T. Respiratory changes before ecdysis. Bull of ARAV, Premiere Issue, 1991:2.

6. Anderson N. Husbandry and clinical evaluation of *Iguana iguana*. Compend Contin Educ Pract Vet, August 1991; 13:1265–1269.

7. Suedmeyer WK. Noninfectious diseases of reptiles. Seminars in Avian and Exotic Pet Medicine, January 1995; 4:56–60.

8. Ritchie B *et al*. Avian medicine: Principles and applications. Lake Worth: Wingers, 1994:458.

9. Raiti P. Veterinary care of the common kingsnake, *Lampropeltis getula*. Bull of ARAV 5:11–18.

Diseases and Treatment of Turtles

▼   ▼   ▼   ▼   ▼   ▼   ▼   ▼

B ECAUSE the box turtle is the species most commonly seen in most veterinarians' practices, this discussion, while applicable to many terrestrial turtles, will focus on this species.

■ COMMON DISEASES

Hypovitaminosis A

Vitamin A deficiency is commonly seen in box turtles that are fed improper diets. The all-meat diet, the "cricket and fruit cocktail" diet, and the "lettuce and carrots diet" are all deficient in Vitamin A (and several other nutrients as well). Vitamin A is needed to maintain epithelial integrity; deficiency produces signs associated with changes in the epidermis. Turtles may show anorexia, lethargy, swelling of the eyes and eyelids (often with a purulent discharge), middle ear abscessation, and respiratory infections (see Fig. 8.1). Differential diagnosis for "conjunctivitis" includes trauma, foreign bodies, helminths, and bacterial/viral/fungal infections; cytologic examination of exudate or the conjunctiva may assist in formulating a diagnosis (1). Chronic deficiency, which shows squamous metaplasia and hyperkeratinization, is more difficult to treat successfully.

Diagnosis is easily made by the clinical signs and the nutritional history.

Treatment includes diet correction and administration of vitamin A; hospitalization is needed for turtles that are anorectic or lethargic, have respiratory infections, and are presumed septic. Injectable vitamin A can be used, but hypervitaminosis A may occur with overdosage. Many veterinarians choose to correct the problem with oral

103
▼

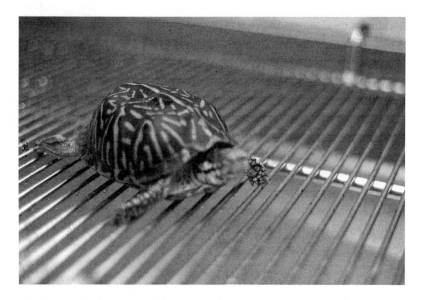

Fig. 8.1 *A box turtle with hypovitaminosis A. Notice the eyelids are closed and swollen. The turtle responded to treatment with vitamin A.*

vitamin A to prevent toxicity that may be seen with injectable vitamin A. The disease can be prevented by feeding the pet a proper diet.

Treatment

1. 0.1 mL Injacom-100 (Roche, 100,000 IU vitamin A/mL)/300 g PO initial dose, then 0.02 mL/week for 2–3 more weeks PO; or 2000 IU/kg Aquasol A parenteral (Armour) SQ once weekly for 4–6 weeks. At 2000 IU/kg, this regimen is usually 0.01–0.02 mL/week. Injacom A has too much vitamin A per mL to give parenterally, as hypervitaminosis A may result (1–3).
2. Slowly improve the diet and have the owner begin using reptile or avian vitamins.
3. Treat secondary problems.

Hypervitaminosis A

This usually iatrogenic disease is caused by treating hypovitaminosis A with the incorrect vitamin A preparation or dosage. The disease is most likely to result from injectable preparations and least likely to occur with oral medication. On rare occasions, an owner may cause hypervitaminosis A by overdosing with daily oral vitamins. Vitamin A toxicity has been seen in turtles treated with injectable vitamin A at a dosage of 5000 IU/kg (1).

Signs include dry or flaky skin (subacute xeroderma; see Fig. 8.2), followed in a few days by a severe loss of skin. The underlying soft tissues and muscles are exposed; lesions typically appear on the limbs, neck, and tail. By the fourteenth day after injection, fluid-filled epidermal blisters appear, which then lift away from the dermis to leave denuded tissue.

Most turtles recover and their skin regenerates. Some animals are so severely affected, however, that infection and tissue fluid loss occur (similar to the situation with third-degree burns). Treatment includes prevention of infections and supportive care.

Treatment

1. Local wound treatment with water-soluble, antimicrobial wet dressings (dilute chlorhexidine diacetate solution, Dakin's

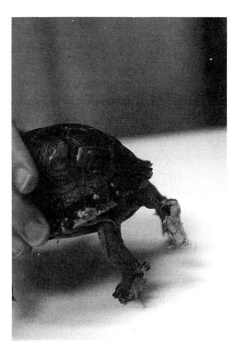

Fig. 8.2 *Flaking of the skin seen in a turtle with hypervitaminosis A.*

solution) or ointments, including Betadine ointment, Furacin ointment, Sulfamylon ointment, or Silvadene cream (my favorite). Opsite spray bandage or Nexaband spray bandage may be used to protect exposed tissue from desiccation and infection. Particulate bedding material should not be used as it adheres to wet dressings and ointments; clean cloth towels, paper towels, and butcher's paper are acceptable instead (2).

2. Surgical debridement if needed.

3. Fluid therapy is necessary when large amounts of denuded tissue are exposed; as much as 75–150 mL/kg may be needed for the first 24–48 hours to ensure renal perfusion (2). Ascorbic acid (100–250 mg/kg IM s.i.d. [3]) and B-complex vitamins (0.25–0.50 mL/kg IM s.i.d. [3]) can be used, or 0.50–1.0 mL of each added to the fluids (2).

4. Blood or plasma may be required in case of extensive tissue loss. Little information is available regarding blood component therapy in reptiles; extrapolation from canine and feline medicine is suggested.

5. Parenteral antibiotics are needed for all but the most minor, localized burns: (see Formulary for an in-depth discussion).
   - Amikacin: 2.5 mg/kg SQ, IM every 72 hours for 5–7 treatments* (2,3)
   - Piperacillin: 200–400 mg/kg IM q24 h* ** (3)
   - Cephalothin: 40–80 mg/kg dd b.i.d.* ** (2)
   - Trimethoprim–Sulfadiazine: 30 mg/kg SQ, IM q24h for 10–14 treatments* (3)

You may want to use enrofloxacin (10 mg/kg IM q24h for 10–14 days) +/− amikacin as your initial antibiotic selection (1,3). (Enrofloxacin may cause anorexia in turtles.)

Respiratory Disease

Respiratory diseases may occur in conjunction with other conditions, including improper diet, vitamin A deficiency, respiratory parasites,

---

* Any of these agents is a rational choice for first-time antibiotic selection. Save enrofloxacin for the more serious cases.
** Combine with amikacin.

or infectious stomatitis. Respiratory disease can be anything as mild as rhinitis or as severe as pneumonia; causative organisms include bacteria (most commonly), fungi, viruses, or parasites. Some tortoises and turtles reportedly have a seasonal clear, serous nasal discharge. This discharge often corresponds to the "allergy" (pollen) season in humans in the area, or may result from excessive dust in the pet's environment. Cytologic examination of the exudate often reveals numerous pollen grains. Assuming the pet is otherwise healthy, no treatment is usually needed; pediatric-strength neosynephrine nose drops may be helpful (Mader, personal communication, 1994).

Lack of a diaphragm prevents active coughing from the air-sac-like lungs of reptiles. The mainstem bronchi and trachea enter the lungs more cranially in reptiles than in mammals. These factors favor the retention of respiratory secretions in the lower airways; simple respiratory infections are, therefore, more prone to developing into pneumonia in reptiles than in mammals. Conversely, muscular anaerobiasis (glycolic respiration) is remarkable in reptiles; they can often survive respiratory infections that would prove fatal to animals lacking anaerobic respiratory capabilities.

Many "simple" respiratory infections in reptiles are actually symptoms of serious lower respiratory disease and may require aggressive treatment. While the prognosis for such infections is always guarded, many turtles will survive *if* appropriate aggressive treatment is instituted. Any turtle that isn't eating, is lethargic, and has severe respiratory signs (e.g., sneezing, wheezing, mucopurulent nasal discharge, dyspnea, open-mouth breathing) should be assumed to have pneumonia until proved otherwise and treated aggressively.

Many of these pets are gravely ill and hospitalization is essential. Hospitalized turtles are kept in an incubator and given fluids and force feeding. Cultures (aerobic and possibly anaerobic) of the respiratory tract are taken, and a tracheal wash and colonic wash are performed to examine for parasites. Injectable antibiotics are administered. Once the turtle begins to improve, the owner can continue antibiotic injections at home. Turtles with "simple" infections can be treated at home with parenteral antibiotics and vitamin A (if needed).

Treatment

1. Maintain hydration with intracoelomic or epicoelomic fluids (15–25 mL/kg for maintenance [2]).
2. Force-feed as needed.
3. Begin antibiotic therapy with the following, pending C&S results: (see Formulary for an in-depth discussion.)
   - Amikacin: 2.5 mg/kg SQ, IM every 72 hours for 5–7 treatments* (2,3)
   - Piperacillin: 200–400 mg/kg IM q24h* ** (3)
   - Cephalothin: 40–80 mg/kg dd b.i.d.* ** (2)
   - Trimethoprim–Sulfadiazine: 30 mg/kg SQ, IM q24h for 10–14 treatments* (3)

   You may want to use enrofloxacin (10 mg/kg IM q24h for 10–14 days) +/− amikacin as your initial antibiotic selection (1,3). (Enrofloxacin may cause anorexia in turtles.)
4. Perform a tracheal wash, cytology, and culture and sensitivity test as needed.
5. Perform a fecal flotation.
6. Maintain a warm (85–90 °F) environment.
7. Nebulization using amikacin or gentamicin may be indicated. Regimens follow those used in birds and mammals. Some veterinarians advocate adding a bronchodilator (Albuterol), cromalyn sodium, and/or acetylcysteine to the nebulizing solution.
8. Oxygen therapy as needed.
9. Furosemide (5 mg/kg IV, IM prn) can reduce respiratory fluids; parenteral fluids should be used concurrently with diuretics (2).
10. Atropine (0.04 mg/kg PO, IV, IM, SQ prn) can be used to dry mucous membranes (2).

Shell Diseases

Aquatic turtles are afflicted with infectious shell diseases more often than land turtles; terrestrial turtles do encounter shell problems (frac-

---

* Any of these agents is a rational choice for first-time antibiotic selection. Save enrofloxacin for the more serious cases.
** Combine with amikacin.

tures) due to trauma, however. Infections, when present, can be bacterial, fungal, or viral (rarely) in origin. Because many infections have similar manifestations, a thorough dermatology workup (culture and sensitivity test, fungal culture, cytology, biopsy) is indicated. Traumatic shell injuries can be the result of dog bites, human injury, or automobile trauma (crushing-type injuries). Shell repair with epoxy may be indicated, as well as parenteral antibiotics for all but superficial traumatic lesions. Shell lesions should be treated as open wounds and only repaired after all evidence of contamination and infection has resolved (2).

Treatment

Shell repair using epoxy resin and fiberglass cloth (2):

1. Carefully debride shell edges; the procedure may be facilitated by using anesthesia (inhalant or ketamine sedation). Butorphanol (0.5–1.0 mg/kg IM postoperatively) or Banamine (1.0 mg/kg IM s.i.d. for 2–3 days maximum (4) should be employed for analgesia.
2. Elevate depressed fragments (small, devitalized fragments less than 3 cm may be discarded).
3. Extensive areas of shell loss will be bridged by the resin-impregnated fiberglass.
4. Use autoclaved round or oval fiberglass patches; the patch should extend for 1.5–3.0 cm beyond the fracture site.
5. Clean the shell with acetone or ether, and allow it to air-dry.
6. Epoxy (such as 5-Minute Epoxy Cement by Devcon, or a similar product) is applied to the periphery of the defect and extended 2 cm beyond the defect. Don't touch the defect and its edges; epoxy interposed between shell fragments will impede bone healing.
7. Apply the first layer of patch over the defect so that the edges of the patch contact the resin; gently work the resin into the patch while it is stretched over the hole. When the resin has polymerized, a *light* coat of resin can be applied to the center of the patch. This coat should moisten only the fabric; resin must not enter the wound.

8. After polymerization of the first layer, several more layers are applied in the same manner until the desired strength and thickness are achieved. Two layers are usually sufficient.

9. After the last coat has polymerized, spray a light coat of Pam vegetable oil coating or an equivalent product over the patch to prevent it from sticking to the cage substrate material.

Complete healing may take two or more years. The patch can be left on for the life of an adult turtle; young growing turtles will need patches removed and replaced as the growth rings expand (possibly every 6 months). Patches can be removed with a rotary file or burr; this material is irritating to the eyes, lungs, and gastrointestinal tract, so appropriate safety measures (e.g., mask, goggles) should be worn.

Abscesses

Diagnosis and treatment of an abscess involves lancing the abscess (often under anesthesia), flushing the cavity, and giving antibiotics (as based on culture and sensitivity tests). Cytological examination of cutaneous and subcutaneous nodules can be performed. Unlike mammalian abscesses, reptilian abscesses contain firm caseated material rather than liquid pus (reptile heterophils lack the lysozymes to degrade and liquefy infectious materials). This structure may complicate the diagnosis of abscesses, although white blood cells and infectious organisms may be seen cytologically. Because the treatment (surgical removal) of the nodule is the same regardless of the cytological diagnosis, I rarely perform aspiration cytology on cutaneous or subcutaneous masses in reptiles unless the owner refuses surgical diagnosis and therapy. Antibiotic therapy could be administered if surgery is refused based on a cytological diagnosis of an abscess, although this treatment is usually unrewarding unless the abscess is opened and debrided.

Care should be taken as some abscesses are caused by zoonotic mycobacterial species.

Abscesses in turtles are often secondary to hypovitaminosis A. A common site for abscessation is the middle ear; vestibular symptoms may persist until the abscess is evacuated. While most abscesses in reptiles contain hard, inspissated pus, the ear abscesses in turtles frequently contain fluid purulent material.

Treatment

1. Debride the abscess; sedation or anesthesia may be needed. Small, superficial abscesses can often be quickly lanced and flushed without sedation or anesthesia.
2. Flush the abscess cavity thoroughly with dilute povidone–iodine solution or chlorhexidine diacetate solution.
3. In contrast to the treatment of abscesses in dogs and cats, abscesses in reptiles are usually sutured (primary closure) due to the high incidence of infection of open wounds (contaminated wounds can, of course, be treated as open wounds). Darkening of the surrounding epidermis may be a possible consequence of healed surgical sites in reptiles.
4. Some veterinarians use a topical antibiotic ointment, such as Silvadene, in the cavity until it heals.
5. Strongly consider gram-staining and/or culturing abscesses, especially those that recur or that do not heal (rule out anaerobic organisms and mycobacteria).
6. Rarely, systemic antibiotics may be needed (see the discussion of infectious stomatitis for antibiotic choices).

Winter Anorexia/Pseudohibernation

Some turtles, particularly those caught in the wild and sold as pets (or caught and kept as pets by owners), may develop winter anorexia. This condition occurs as the days become shorter and cooler. The temperature is not cold enough to encourage true hibernation; the cooler temperatures encourage anorexia, but the metabolic rate of the turtle does not slow sufficiently and it begins to starve. Treatment involves allowing the pet to hibernate (if it is in good health and if it has not been anorectic for too long) or encouraging the turtle to eat by artificially increasing daylight. Treat other problems (hypovitaminosis A and respiratory tract infections) concurrently. A brief discussion of hibernation follows.

Hibernation (4)

If given the opportunity, turtles will hibernate. Hibernation does not appear to be necessary (this topic is an area of controversy), but some owners wish to provide suitable conditions for hibernating. Hibernation is necessary for adequate reproduction, however. If the temperature of the environment stays warm, some turtles may stop eating in the fall while others continue feeding and skip hibernation. Hibernation is very stressful, and subclinical illnesses can manifest themselves during hibernation. *Only turtles that are in good health should be allowed to hibernate, so a thorough examination and appropriate laboratory tests are essential prior to hibernation!*

If hibernation occurs, it usually begins in the fall (September or October). As the temperature drops—especially if the cage temperature cools—the turtle may decrease its appetite. At this time, food (but not water) should be withheld for 1–2 weeks and the temperature maintained at 70–80°F. This process will allow the turtle the chance to eliminate and clear its gastrointestinal tract. After this period, the external heat source is removed for a week and the turtle allowed to remain at room temperature (60–70°F). The turtle can then be placed in its hibernating compartment (hibernaculum).

The hibernaculum should have dim light and a temperature of 50–60°F. An occasional drop to 45°F is acceptable. Temperatures that persist above 60°F are not cool enough for true hibernation and allow the turtle to increase its metabolism and slowly starve ("pseudohibernation"). Temperatures below 45°F are detrimental as well. For its own safety, the turtle should not be allowed to hibernate outdoors where temperature and predators can't be controlled.

The hibernaculum should have a foot of humid peat-based potting soil and a 3–6 in. layer of shredded newspaper or leaves or hay on top, allowing the turtle to burrow. The soil should remain damp, but not wet, to prevent the turtle from dehydrating. A small water bowl should be present to offer humidity and prevent dehydration. As a rule, turtles will hibernate for 3–5 months. Any turtle that appears ill during hibernation (it should be checked at least weekly) should be immediately examined. Pneumonia is often seen during hibernation; signs of this disease include nasal discharge, mucus in the mouth, and gurgling respiratory noises.

At the end of hibernation (early spring), the turtle should be placed back into its regular cage and the temperature slowly warmed to the normal range over a 1-week period. Food should then be offered.

Treatment

1. Use full-spectrum lights; increase the photoperiod by 1/2 hour per week until 14 hours of light per day are reached. Do not let natural light (daylight) interfere with this process (put the cage in a closet or windowless room) (1,5).

2. Ensure proper environmental temperature (75–85 °F) (1,6).

■ **LESS COMMON CONDITIONS**

Infectious Stomatitis

Infectious stomatitis ("mouth rot"), which is almost always caused by bacteria, is rarely diagnosed in chelonians. Most cases may look severe, but often require only topical treatment. While many bacteria can cause the problem, *Pseudomonas* and *Aeromonas* are the most common culprits. Infectious stomatitis is generally considered to be a secondary disease, as *Pseudomonas* and *Aeromonas* are often normally present in a reptile's environment and body. A dirty environment is one cause of the condition. Other stressors that can cause infectious stomatitis include internal parasites, poor diet, improper environment and improper environmental temperature, shipping (as when a pet is brought into an owner's home after purchase), too little or too much handling, a too humid or too dry cage, and almost any other stress. The stress isn't always identified, but the pet should undergo a thorough diagnostic workup (treat the pet, not the disease!).

Early symptoms that often go unnoticed by owners include petechial hemorrhages inside the oral cavity. These signs may be seen during a routine physical examination on an otherwise asymptomatic turtle or in the oral cavity of a turtle presented for another medical problem. Don't overlook these early lesions; begin treatment if they are detected. The later stage of the disease reveals a large amount of frothy, bubbly mucus or a "cottage cheese" type of material. Many animals in the later stages are anorectic and lethargic.

Diagnosis is fairly easy and is made by observation of the oral cavity. All obvious cases as well as suspected cases (where the amount or character of the mucus seems abnormal or where petechial hemorrhages are seen) of mouth rot should be cultured. *Pseudomonas* and *Aeromonas* are often found in many normal reptiles, so their presence on a culture doesn't always mean the pet has or will develop mouth rot. Any heavy growth on a culture should probably be treated, however.

Treatment varies with the severity of the disease. Compared with iguanas and snakes, turtles are rarely afflicted with this disease. Many cases in turtles appear severe but usually no parenteral treatment is needed; in most instances, infectious stomatitis in turtles can be treated by correcting underlying problems (parasites, hypo-vita-minosis A) and using topical antibacterial rinses. Turtles that are anorectic and lethargic need to be hospitalized. During hospital-ization, these severely ill patients are given fluids, kept warm in an incubator, and force-fed.

While the practitioner awaits the culture results, turtles with severe stomatitis and septicemia are started on injectable antibiotics. The oral cavity is treated with a topical medication, such as dilute povidone–iodine, chlorhexidinediacetate, hydrogen peroxide, and/ or Silvadene. Atropine injections are given if the mucus is thick; many veterinarians feel that atropine helps to thin the mucus and allow for easier removal by the animal's body. Vitamin B complex injections are administered. Vitamin C also seems to help clinically in mouth rot.

The prognosis of mouth rot depends upon several factors. Because the condition is mild and requires only topical treatment in most turtles, the prognosis is good to excellent. If the animal is still eating and active, the prognosis is good. If the disease is diagnosed early, when only the petechial hemorrhages are seen, the prognosis is also very good. Animals that haven't eaten in several days or weeks, are weak and depressed, and have large amounts of mucus in their oral cavities are often septic and have a much poorer chance of recovery. Secondary problems, such as internal parasites, also need to be addressed. Once the animal has recovered, the diet is slowly corrected and the environment is changed.

Treatment (Mild Cases)

Unlike with most reptiles, infectious stomatitis occurs only rarely in turtles and is usually mild. Most cases require only topical therapy. Parenteral antibiotics are listed for those extremely rare cases where the infection is especially severe (2).

1. Culture and sensitivity test of the oral cavity.
2. Oral therapy to include topical rinses performed as follows:
   - Dilute chlorhexidine diacetate solution (0.25–1.0%) (2)
   - Dilute povidone–iodine solution (1%) (2)
   - Acetic acid (vinegar) (dilute to a 0.5% solution) (2)
   - Hydrogen peroxide

   Rinses are given b.i.d.; the mouth is rinsed with plain water after the rinses are used. Alternating rinses (i.e., chlorhexidine day 1, peroxide day 2, acetic acid day 3, with the regimen repeated for the duration of treatment) may be helpful. You may decide to alternate rinses as follows: chlorhexidine in the morning, peroxide in the evening, and so on. *Wear eye protection (goggles) and have clients do the same when rinsing the oral cavity!*
3. Topical Silvadene.

Treatment (Severe Cases)

1. In addition to the treatment listed for mild cases, severely ill pets need hospitalization with fluid therapy, incubation, and force feeding.
2. Begin antibiotic therapy with the following, pending C&S results: (see Formulary for an in-depth discussion).
   - Amikacin: 2.5 mg/kg SQ, IM every 72 hours for 5–7 treatments* (2,3)
   - Piperacillin: 200–400 mg/kg IM q24h* ** (3)
   - Cephalothin: 40–80 mg/kg dd b.i.d.* ** (2)

---

*Any of these agents is a rational choice for first-time antibiotic selection. Save enrofloxacin for the more serious cases.
**Combine with amikacin.

- Trimethoprim–Sulfadiazine: 30 mg/kg SQ, IM q24h for 10–14 treatments* (3)

Enrofloxacin +/− amikacin can be used as your initial antibiotic selection in especially weakened or septic animals at 10 mg/kg IM q24h for 10–14 days (1,3). (Enrofloxacin may cause anorexia in turtles.)

Many veterinarians recommend parenteral fluids in any reptile receiving aminoglycosides, and to a lesser extent piperacillin and cephalosporins, to prevent renal damage.

For cases that don't respond to appropriate antimicrobial therapy, consider an anaerobic infection. Perform an anaerobic culture and treat with metronidazole, clindamycin, or tetracycline. Anaerobes may account for up to 50% of reptile "infections."

Metabolic Bone Disease

Metabolic bone disease—also called nutritional osteodystrophy, nutritional secondary hyperparathyroidism, or rubber jaw—is rarely seen in turtles. It is not as prevalent as in iguanas. Owners typically present turtles with signs of vitamin A deficiency and/or respiratory diseases before metabolic bone disease has a chance to occur (or at least before signs are detected). This condition may also be diagnosed less often in turtles because clinical signs of metabolic bone disease differ from the signs seen in iguanas. You may be treating a turtle that actually has metabolic bone disease but isn't showing signs of this problem at the time of presentation; correcting the diet (as is needed with vitamin A deficiency) will correct the metabolic bone disease before the condition becomes clinically apparent. The condition usually results from a lack of calcium and/or vitamin D_3 in the diet; renal, hepatic, thyroid, or parathyroid disease may also cause this disease.

Even though the blood calcium level usually remains normal during affliction, the animal can still show signs of illness. Symptoms include appendicular fractures and gross deformities of the carapace (dorsal shell) and plastron (ventral shell). The lateral scutes (plates) of

---

* Any of these agents is a rational choice for first-time antibiotic selection. Save enrofloxacin for the more serious cases.

the carapacial–plastral bridge expand and grow dorsoventrally; the shells assume a spherical shape.

If the turtle is still active and eating, the prognosis is better. A complete physical examination is needed before treating metabolic bone disease. Often, these animals also have vitamin A deficiency, and possibly infectious stomatitis, septicemia, or internal parasites. A thorough examination and radiographs (if needed) can provide a wealth of prognostic information. As always, "treat the pet, not the disease." Individuals with parasites, infectious stomatitis, or other problems need these issues addressed as well as the metabolic bone disease.

Turtles that are still active and eating can be treated at home. Injections of calcium gluconate (see the section on "Treatment") are given intracoelomically* by the owner (most owners can easily be taught to perform this procedure), or oral calcium can be used. Ultraviolet light is supplied as well. Often, a vitamin injection is given. The owner should be instructed to begin changing the diet *slowly*. The easiest way to make this change is by adding a small amount of a balanced vegetable mixture (see chapter 4) and decreasing the regular diet by about 10% per week. Although the diet must eventually be changed, it's acceptable if the turtle refuses to eat the new diet at first. It's more important for the pet to eat a bad diet than nothing at all. Because the turtle is receiving concomitant treatment with injectable or oral calcium and UV light, it can improve despite the bad diet. Recovery, if it occurs, typically occurs after 4–6 weeks of injections. Owners should be instructed to remove all objects from the cage except the food and water bowls.

Turtles that are lethargic and anorectic have a guarded prognosis, but treatment should always be offered. Compared with other reptiles, turtles—even those affected with serious disease conditions—rarely die. Severely ill turtles need hospitalization in which they are placed in an incubator and given intracoelomic fluids. Force feeding is used to stimulate appetite and to prevent a negative nitrogen balance and catabolic state. If improvement (increased activ-

---

Intracoelomic is the correct term because turtles lack a diaphragm and, therefore, a peritoneal cavity. Some authors use the term *intraperitoneal* interchangeably with *intracoelomic*.

ity and resumption of feeding) occurs, it usually is seen within 2–3 days of intensive care.

Treatment (Mild Cases)

1. Calcium injections. Several regimens exist:
   - 10% calcium gluconate intracoelomically, 100 mg/mL, 500 mg/kg weekly for 4–6 weeks* (2,6)
   - Calphosan 0.5–1.0 mL/kg (50–100 mg/kg) IM weekly for 4–6 weeks* (7)
   - Oral calcium (Neo-Calglucon) at 1.0 mL/kg (23 mg/kg) b.i.d. (8)
2. Dietary correction.
3. UV light.
4. Remove any cage objects that might injure the pet.
5. B-complex vitamin injection: 0.25–0.50 mL/kg (once is usually adequate) (3)
6. Injacom-100: Dose at 100 IU vitamin D_3/kg SQ, two doses one week apart (9).
7. Mineral supplementation. Osteoform tablets are acceptable; dose at 200 IU D_3/kg/week (6). The tablets should be crushed, and the correct amount sprinkled on the food weekly. After 2–4 months, you can switch to a supplement containing only calcium to avoid hypervitaminosis D. As a rule, a daily sprinkling of a calcium supplement is adequate. The amount to sprinkle on the food is equivalent to the *light* salting a person would give his or her own food.
8. Vitamin supplementation. A light sprinkling of a good bird or reptile vitamin 1–2 times each week is adequate.

Treatment (Severe Cases)

1. Intracoelomic injections of fluids at 15–25 mL/kg/day (1–3% of body weight/day) for maintenance (2).
2. Incubation at 85–90 °F.

---

*The duration of 4–6 weeks is arbitrary. Most pets respond within this period of time. If the turtle is responding but not yet "cured," the treatment can be extended as needed.

An alternative regimen in iguanas that may prove useful in severely affected turtles (but has not been tried by the author or reported in the literature) involves the use of calcitonin (8):

1. Start calcium glubionate (Neo-Calglucon syrup, USP) at 1 mL/kg (23 mg/kg) PO q12h on the first visit. 10% Calcium gluconate (100 mg/kg IM q6h prn for up to 24 hours) can be given if hypocalcemic tetany is present. (I often give an initial ICe injection of 10% calcium gluconate at 500 mg/kg on the first visit.) The Neocalglucon is often continued for more than a year (given s.i.d. after stabilization) when treating iguanas; no studies have been done using this drug or treatment regimen in turtles.

2. Injacom-100 (dosed at 1000 IU vitamin D_3/kg) IM once weekly for two treatments.

3. If the turtle is normocalcemic, give calcitonin* (Miacalin, Schering Plough, Kenilworth, New Jersey, or Calcimar) at 50 IU/kg IM once weekly at the week 2 and 3 visits. (If serum calcium levels are unknown, no problems should arise when using calcitonin as long as the Neocalglucon has been given as directed.)

External Parasites

External parasites are rarely seen in reptiles compared with dogs and cats. See chapter 9 for a complete discussion of this topic.

Internal Parasites

Internal parasites are commonly seen in turtles. See chapter 9 for a complete discussion of this topic.

Cystic Calculi

Cystic calculi occur when minerals from the diet form crystals that then form stones. Usually these stones are composed of uric

---

*Calcitonin has been used in iguanas for metabolic bone disease; it may or may not be effective or harmful in turtles. Veterinarians should inform owners that this treatment is experimental.

acid, which typically results from a diet that contains too much protein.

Blood in the droppings can be a sign of cystic calculi, as can a palpable abdominal mass. Diagnosis is made by physical examination and radiography. Surgical removal of the stones is needed, as is fluid therapy to prevent kidney damage; diet should be corrected to prevent reoccurrence. Turtles with this condition are often on diets too high in animal protein, such as dog or cat food. Switching them to a diet high in plant protein is essential.

Treatment

1. Cystotomy (either a flank approach or a transplastral approach is advocated).
2. Fluids prn (15–25 mL/kg/day for maintenance [2]).
3. Dietary correction.
4. Antibiotics if needed, based on C&S.

Organ Failure

As with so many pets, renal and hepatic failure can be seen in turtles. The turtles so affected are usually older pets. As in mammals, chronic renal and hepatic failure is not reversible. The problem is often not detected until it's too late. Organ failure may result from gout, infections, tumors, or incorrect diets. Treatment, when attempted, involves aggressive fluid therapy and antibiotics. Lactulose and phosphate binders may be tried, with dosages extrapolated from mammalian and avian regimens.

Treatment

1. Often detected in end-stage organ failure, so prognosis is poor to grave.
2. Fluids and force feeding.
3. Antibiotics (avoid nephrotoxic antibiotics).

Salmonella

While box turtles are infamous for this condition, any reptile can carry the *Salmonella* bacterium. Because of the high prevalence in box turtles, legislation was enacted that made it illegal to sell turtles with a shell diameter under 4 inches—a size chosen as the largest turtle that a child can place into his or her mouth! This restriction has greatly reduced the occurrence of *Salmonella* in children.

Salmonella, a gram-negative bacterium, can cause severe gastrointestinal disease or septicemia in reptiles and their owners. Many animals and people are asymptomatic carriers. Most pet reptiles probably carry *Salmonella* as a part of their normal enteric flora, acting as asymptomatic carriers. True infection may occur when pets are stressed, resulting in an impaired immune system, which allows the normal flora to become pathogenic (2). *Salmonella* infection can cause clinical disease in pet reptiles. Clinical signs include acute enteritis and septicemia, pneumonia, coelomitis, hypovolemic shock, and death (2). The feces of clinically ill reptiles may contain mucus, or blood, and be colored green–gray (2).

Prevention, through proper hygiene, is the best way to control the disease. Because most animals that carry the bacterium aren't ill, they require no treatment (treating carriers often fails to eradicate the organism).

Dystocia

Dystocia, or egg-binding, is occasionally encountered in turtles. Unlike mammals, dystocia is often *not* a medical emergency; even with medical treatment, reptiles may not pass any retained eggs for a few days and still survive with no ill effects. An examination or treatment should not be delayed, however, as early diagnosis and treatment improves the prognosis. Many owners don't detect early signs of dystocia (often the sex of the reptile isn't known even to the owner); the pet may not be examined until later in the course of the condition, when the problem may have become an emergency, requiring hospitalization and all of the supportive care required by any "sick" reptile.

If the animal is known to be female, dystocia is more easily diagnosed. Often one or several eggs have already been passed, and the pet continues to strain as if trying to pass the remaining eggs. If no eggs have been passed, diagnosis is more difficult. Abdominal palpation may allow detection of the eggs; radiographs may be necessary for a diagnosis. Abdomen is obviously swollen. Owners may complain of polyuria, diarrhea, or blood in the droppings. Definitive diagnosis requires radiographs; chelonians' eggs have a calcified outer shell.

The cause of dystocia is often unknown. Poor diet, incorrect environmental temperature, improper nesting site, and internal disease are all contributing factors. For some reason, the uterus fails to expel the egg, which becomes stuck. Occasionally, the egg is too large to pass through the cloaca, resulting in dystocia.

Treatment is to relieve the dystocia and allow the turtle to pass the eggs. As with dogs and cats with dystocia, several treatment options are available.

Treatment

1. For eggs that are near the cloaca, lubrication of the cloaca and gentle manipulation can be tried first.
2. If lubrication and manipulation fail to correct the situation, calcium gluconate or lactate (10–50 mg/kg [3]) or calcium glycerophosphate and lactate (Calphosan, 1.0–2.5 mL/kg [100–250 mg/kg] [3]) and oxytocin (1–10 units [3,4]) IM are tried next. (Oxytocin at 1–2 IU/kg IM in the front or rear legs, with or without calcium, is usually effective in resolving dystocia in chelonians [9].) The turtle can be returned to the owner with instructions to keep it quiet, avoid handling, and place the turtle in a warm environment (85°F). Most turtles will pass eggs within 24–72 hours. Ovacentesis can be used prior to oxytocin and calcium, especially if the eggs appear enlarged (usually due to egg death and decomposition). Dehydration should be corrected prior to using ecbolic agents.
3. If no eggs are passed after 24–72 hours, a repeat dose of calcium and oxytocin can be administered. Surgical removal may be indicated at this point.
4. Alternatively, Calphosan (0.2–0.5 mL/kg [20–50 mg/kg] IM or SQ) followed by arginine vasotocin (0.01–1.0 µm/kg IV or IP) can be used (8). Inderal (1.0 µg/g) followed by vasotocin (500 ng/g [10]) has also been reported. The literature has suggested greater efficacy with this protocol than with calcium and oxytocin; arginine vasotocin is expensive, however, and is not currently available except for research purposes.

5.   Ovariohysterectomy may be indicated. Some veterinarians recommend hysterectomy rather than ovariohysterectomy.

For turtles that are obviously ill at the time of presentation, supportive care is needed. In addition, surgical intervention (either a flank approach or a transplastral incision) can be considered as a first option after the pet is stabilized.

Many practitioners feel that oxytocin, especially if used as the sole agent, is unsuccessful in treating dystocia in reptiles. However, oxytocin is usually effective in chelonians. Oxytocin requires a hydrated uterine mucosa; prolonged egg retention results in a greater adherence of the uterine mucosa to the eggs as a result of mucosal dehydration. Some veterinarians feel that calcium is not useful prior to oxytocin injection but can be administered after several oxytocin injections. Multiple doses of oxytocin can result in uterine rupture if the etiology of the dystocia is enlarged eggs. Many doctors report success with a combination of calcium and arginine vasotocin. As with mammalian dystocia, treatment varies by practitioner and the treatment listed here is intended to serve as only a guideline.

Gastrointestinal Obstruction

Obstructions of the gastrointestinal tract can occur in turtles as the result of heavy parasite burdens (typically roundworms), foreign bodies (usually in young turtles), cage bedding (especially if sand, shells, or corncob is used), or neoplasia. Signs are nonspecific but may include abdominal distention with tympany. Radiographs are needed to confirm obstructions and associated gaseous distention and ileus. Surgical intervention is often required to correct the problem.

Treatment
1.   Supportive care prn.
2.   Exploratory laparotomy.

Cloacal Prolapse

Cloacal prolapse can occur secondary to chronic straining, inflammation, infection, parasites, and dystocia. It rarely occurs idiopathically. Repair is conducted under light sedation or isoflurane anesthesia.

The prolapse can be replaced (often with a pursestring or transverse suture) or excised (with electrosurgery being used to control bleeding). Chronic prolapses require a cloacapexy.

Treatment

1. In mild cases, cleaning, lubrication, and replacement (with pursestring or transverse suture if needed) may work. Lidocaine gel, 50% dextrose, or glycerin may reduce the swelling. A linear cloacal incision (similar to an episiotomy) may reduce the swelling. A fecal examination can rule out internal parasites.
2. Amputation (using electrosurgery if needed) if replacement is not feasible. The procedure is not bloody and is fairly straightforward. Incise a small amount of tissue with a scalpel and suture that section before proceeding to the next section of tissue.
3. Cloacapexy in cases of chronic prolapse.

Penile Prolapse

Prolapse of the penis is occasionally encountered. Proposed etiologies include osteodystrophy; bacterial, parasitic, or fungal infections; trauma while breeding; and neurogenic defects of the penile or cloacal musculature. Treatment is similar to that used for cloacal prolapse. Differential diagnosis includes a prolapsed cloaca, intestine, and bladder.

Treatment

1. In mild cases, cleaning, lubrication, and replacement (with pursestring suture if needed) may work. Preparation H, lidocaine gel, or 50% dextrose may reduce swelling.
2. Amputation (electrosurgically) is carried out if replacement is not feasible.

Septicemia

Septicemia, usually bacterial in nature, can result as a direct infection of the blood or after a localized infection spreads hematogenously.

Septic animals are gravely ill and require hospitalization and intensive therapy.

Septic turtles are anorectic and lethargic, and often have pinpoint hemorrhagic areas on their mucous membranes.

Supportive care is similar to that given to turtles hospitalized for respiratory infections.

Treatment

1. Maintain hydration with intracoelomic or epicoelomic fluids, 15–25 mL/kg/day for maintenance (2).
2. Force-feed as needed.
3. Begin antibiotic therapy with the following, pending C&S results: (see Formulary for an in-depth discussion.)
    *   Amikacin: 2.5 mg/kg SQ, IM every 72 hours for 5–7 treatments* (2,3)
    *   Piperacillin: 200–400 mg/kg IM q24h* ** (3)
    *   Cephalothin: 40–80 mg/kg dd b.i.d.* ** (2)
    *   Trimethoprim–Sulfadiazine: 30 mg/kg SQ, IM q24h for 10–14 treatments* (3)
    You may want to use enrofloxacin (10 mg/kg IM q24h for 10–14 days) +/− amikacin as your initial antibiotic selection (1,3).
4. Perform a tracheal wash, cytology, and culture and sensitivity test as needed.
5. Perform a fecal flotation.
6. Maintain a warm (85–90 °F) environment.

Regurgitation

Vomiting and regurgitation are rarely encountered medical problems in reptiles. When seen, a guarded to poor prognosis is warranted, especially in turtles. Causes include improper environmental temperature, infectious disease, metabolic disease, intoxications, parasites, foreign bodies, ulcerative disease, ingestion of putrefied or

---

*Any of these agents is a rational choice for first-time antibiotic selection. Save enrofloxacin for the more serious cases.
**Combine with amikacin.

contaminated (spoiled) food, abscesses, and neoplasia. Handling a turtle soon after eating may occasionally result in regurgitation. A thorough diagnostic array of tests is often needed to determine the cause; a gastric lavage and microscopic examination are required in most cases. Treatment depends upon the cause of the condition. Vomiting and regurgitation are not diseases themselves, but serious signs of disease.

Diarrhea

True diarrhea is rare in reptiles. What most owners consider diarrhea is, in fact, polyuria. A fecal examination is always indicated in any pet with diarrhea, as often internal parasites are the culprits. Diet may also be a cause, particularly if large amounts of fruit are fed to the pet. Bacteria (usually gram-negative pathogens) are also a possible cause of diarrhea in reptiles. Blood profiles, cytological examination and cultures of a colonic and/or gastric lavage, and radiographs may be necessary to determine a cause for the diarrhea. As with vomiting, diarrhea is a clinical sign and not a disease.

Myiasis

Myiasis is caused by deposition of first instar larvae (usually of *Calliphora* or *Sarcophagidea* flies) on open wounds, including shell wounds. A crusty black discharge at the skin–shell margin can be a sign of myiasis. Larval development takes 42–55 days. Treatment involves removal of the larvae and wound flushing.

Treatment

1. Remove maggots (anesthesia or sedation is occasionally needed).
2. Flush wound with dilute chlorhexidine diacetate solution or povidone–iodine solution.
3. Topical or systemic antibiotics are needed on rare occasions.
4. Inspect the turtle for other areas of infestation.

Overgrown Maxilla

Keratinized maxillary tissue may overgrow in chelonians, particularly those that are fed soft diets and that are not allowed to forage for food. These parts can be filed (under anesthesia) if they are not severely overgrown; fractures can be repaired with epoxy in the same way as shell repairs.

Mandibular overgrowths may be more challenging, as malocclusion may occasionally be present. Radiographs may be necessary to determine the amount of tissue to be trimmed. Because trimming may involve entry into the bony cavities (medullary cavity, marrow), use of aseptic technique is important. Epoxy can be applied as needed; severe "beak" malocclusions can be handled "orthodontically" as with avian patients.

Gout

In reptiles, uric acid is the end-product of protein metabolism and is excreted by the renal tubules. Hyperuricemia occurs when the kidneys are unable to filter uric acid from the blood; as a result, urates deposit in various body sites. Hyperuricemia can develop secondary to dehydration, high-protein diets, renal failure, and antibiotic (specifically aminoglycoside) usage (2,11). In one study in snakes, postprandial uric acid levels peaked (10–18 mg/dL) by the fourth day after feeding; levels returned to normal within 2 weeks after feeding (12). The same phenomenon may occur in other reptiles. Uric acid levels should be evaluated in light of diet and time of recent feeding.

While not reported in turtles, visceral and articular gout may also be seen in tortoises and therefore has been included in this chapter. Symptoms depend upon the site affected. Appendicular gout, which causes lameness and swelling, is less common than visceral gout (to which the liver, kidney, spleen, and pericardium are predisposed). Subcutaneous and sublingual uric acid deposits may also be seen in gout; obstipation can be seen if the intestines are involved. Joint aspirates may reveal uric acid crystals, confirming a diagnosis. Radiographs may reveal calcified tophi and/or joint swelling. Calcification of internal organs may be visible radiographically in visceral gout. A common cause is an incorrect diet (containing dog or cat food or excessive amounts of animal-based protein). Dietary correction is needed; treatment is supportive. Allopurinol can be tried as a therapy, but reportedly has poor success.

Treatment

1. Supportive (e.g., fluids).
2. Allopurinol.*
3. Avoid nephrotoxic drugs.
4. Dietary correction.

■ **REFERENCES**

1. Boyer T. Common problems of box turtles (*Terrapene spp.*) in captivity. Bull of ARAV 2:9–16.
2. Frye F. Reptile care: An atlas of diseases and treatments, Vols. I and II. Neptune City, NJ: TFH, 1991.
3. Jenkins J. Medical management of reptile patients. Compend Contin Educ Pract Vet, June 1991; 13:980–988.
4. Messonnier SP. Exotic pets: A veterinary guide for owners. Plano, Texas: Wordware, 1995.
5. Boyer T. Box turtle care. Bull of ARAV 2:14–16.
6. Boyer T. Common problems and treatment of green iguanas (*Iguana iguana*). Bull of ARAV, Premiere Issue:8–11.
7. Anderson N. Husbandry and clinical evaluation of *Iguana iguana*. Compend Contin Educ Pract Vet, August 1991; 13:1265–1269.
8. Mader D. Use of calcitonin in green iguanas, *Iguana iguana*, with metabolic bone disease. Bull of ARAV 3:5.
9. Boyer T. Emergency care of reptiles. Seminars in avian and exotic pet medicine, October 1994; 4:210–216.
10. Suedmeyer WK. Noninfectious diseases of reptiles. Seminars in avian and exotic pet medicine, January 1995; 4:56–60.
11. Ritchie B *et al.* Avian medicine: Principles and applications. Lake Worth: Wingers, 1994:458.
12. Raiti P. Veterinary care of the common kingsnake, *Lampropeltis getula*. Bull of ARAV 5:11–18.

---

*Allopurinol was ineffective in the few cases where it was used (2). A trial therapy may be indicated; an empirical dose (avian dose) uses one 100 mg tablet that is crushed in 10 mL of water; one drop of this mixture is given per 30 g of body weight q.i.d. (12). A dosage of 20 mg/kg PO s.i.d. for 2 weeks in turtles and snakes has been suggested; this same regimen may be effective in iguanas (12).

Parasites

▼ ▼ ▼ ▼ ▼ ▼ ▼ ▼

REPTILES can be infected by a variety of internal or external parasites. Animals in the wild are affected more frequently than domestically raised pets. All reptiles should have a fresh fecal sample (collected via a colonic wash) examined yearly for internal parasites. This chapter will present a quick overview of some commonly seen parasites of reptiles. A parasitology reference text should be consulted for a more thorough discussion of the life cycles of individual parasites.

■ EXTERNAL PARASITES

Iguanas

Ticks (*Amblyomma* and *Ixodes* spp., among others) and mites (*Hirstiella* spp.) can be encountered in iguanas, although they are more common in animals captured in the wild. These parasites ingest blood and may cause serious debilitation in reptiles. In addition, they may be responsible for spreading diseases such as infectious stomatitis. Diagnosis is by observation of the parasite.

Snakes

Ticks (*Amblyomma* and *Ixodes* spp., among others) and mites (*Ophionyssus natricis*, the common snake mite, and *Mabuyonyssus* spp., which parasitize the lungs and trachea) can be encountered in snakes, although they are more common in animals captured in the wild. These parasites ingest blood and may cause serious debilitation in reptiles. They may also spread diseases such as infectious stomatitis. Diagnosis is by observation of the parasite.

Turtles

Ticks (*Amblyomma* and *Ixodes* spp., among others) and fly larvae (*Calliphora* flesh flies, commonly called blowflies, which cause myiasis) can be encountered in turtles, although they are more common in animals captured in the wild. The ticks ingest blood and may cause serious debilitation in reptiles. In addition, they may be responsible for spreading diseases such as infectious stomatitis. Diagnosis is by observation of the parasite (see chapter 8 on turtle diseases for a complete discussion of myiasis).

Treatment of Mites and Ticks

1. Ivermectin: 0.2 mg/kg SQ, IM, PO; repeat in 14 days (my preferred treatment). *This treatment is contraindicated in animals who have or will be treated with diazepam within 10 days, and in turtles and tortoises. It may cause skin discoloration if given SQ (1,2).*

    For snakes, ivermectin spray can be prepared by mixing 0.5 mL of ivermectin (1% bovine product) with 1 liter of water and then directly spraying the animal. Topical treatment kills the mites within 2 hours; it is not necessary to remove residual ivermectin from the snake (3).

2. Dichlorvos strip: Hung within 6 in. of the cage (not in it) for 3 days, and then removed for 7 days. This regimen is repeated four times (4). These strips can be toxic to reptiles and people.

3. Pyrethrin kitten spray: After thoroughly disinfecting the cage, bowls, and other cage objects (e.g., hiding box), spray the cage only. Three days later, spray the cage and tail of the pet; if no signs of toxicity are noted, spray the entire cage and lizard, turtle, or snake *lightly* every 3 days for 3 weeks. You can also spray a cloth and then rub the pet with the cloth (4).

    Mader has used Durakyl, (Dum Pharmaceuticals, Miami, FL) which contains 0.35% Resmethrin, effectively and safely in treating reptiles with mite infestations (5).

    Snake mites have been successfully treated using permectrin spray (Permectrin II, Bio-Ceutic). The stock compound was diluted to a 1% solution with tap water and applied to snakes using a spray bottle. After disinfecting the cage, bowls, and hiding boxes with Roccal-D (Winthrop Laboratories), the cage, water bowls, and hiding boxes were thoroughly sprayed; excess spray was removed with paper towel. The snake was lightly sprayed, excess spray was wiped with a paper towel, and the snake was placed in a clean holding cage for 24 hours. The procedure was repeated in 10 days, and again in 10 days if third treatment was needed. The snake was washed with water 1 day prior to treatment. Only one toxic reaction was seen in a snake treated 10 days earlier with 2% trichlorfon solution.

The snake, which exhibited convulsions, ataxia, and open-mouth breathing, was treated with fluids and corticosteroids. Complete recovery occurred within 5 days (3).

I have observed one toxic reaction in a small infant king-snake that was sprayed with pyrethrin flea spray (approved for cats). The snake exhibited tremors and bizarre behavior immediately after being sprayed. The spray was immediately removed with careful rinsing of the snake with soap and water; one injection of diazepam was given IM. The snake was placed in a dark cage; the behavior lessened but was still present. The behavior was worse when the room lights were turned on and the snake was handled (i.e., worse signs appeared when the snake was stimulated). No other treatment was instituted, and the snake recovered within 24 hours.

Pyrethrin-type sprays should be used cautiously in snakes and other reptiles; pyrethroid products may be safer than pyrethrin products.

4. Sevin Dust (5% carbaryl): For treating snake mites. Remove the snake from the cage. Wash the cage and its furnishings with soap and water, rinse, wash with 5% bleach, rinse, and dry thoroughly. Sprinkle Sevin Dust in the cage. Return only the snake to the cage for 24 hours. Remove the snake, clean and dry the cage, wipe excess dust off of the snake, and then return the snake and the furnishings to the cage. Repeat the procedure in 2 weeks.

Another successful protocol with carbaryl dust involves dusting the snake and leaving the powder on for 30 minutes. The snake is then washed with tap water. The cage must also be disinfected (3).

5. Trichlorfon spray (Trichlorfon pour-on cattle insecticide, Chem-Tronics, Inc., Leavenworth, Kansas) diluted to 0.15% (8 mL of stock 8% solution with 400 mL of water): The cage and bowls, toys, and other furnishings are cleaned with 3% bleach and dried. Newspaper is used for the substrate. The entire set-up is lightly sprayed with the 0.15% Trichlorfon solution and allowed to dry *before* replacing the reptile. The reptile is then *lightly* sprayed. Water is withheld for 24 hours so that the pet doesn't accidentally soak and ingest the Trichlorfon. Repeat the process in 2 weeks. Note that the diluted solution remains stable for about 1 month (6).

Treatment failures most commonly result as a failure to treat the environment properly. When using only ivermectin, the cage bedding must be replaced and the cage cleaned. Ivermectin is *contraindicated in turtles* and in any animal that has been, or will be, treated with diazepam or Telazol within 10 days of the insecticide treatment. Treat all pets in contact with the affected animal regardless of the presence of parasites on cagemates.

■ **INTERNAL PARASITES**

It is important to differentiate parasites of prey (rodents) from parasites of reptiles. Often, the pet is inadvertently treated for prey parasites or pseudoparasites. Always inquire about the diet being fed to the pet. In addition, with all parasitic diseases, the environment should be disinfected (usually dilute chlorine bleach, 1 part to 20–30 parts of water, is acceptable).

Protozoa

1. *Entamoeba invadens* (snakes, iguanas, is turtles) is rare in turtles, and most common in snakes. Signs include regurgitation (often undigested food) or severe diarrhea that may contain blood or bile-tinged green mucus or intestinal mucosal

remnants. Hepatic lesions may be present at necropsy, but renal lesions are rarely found.

Entamoeba invadens can cause human and animal meningoencephalitis. Experimentally, its incubation period is 12–32 days; natural infection probably falls within this range. It is diagnosed by fecal examination or histopathology; it is indistinguishable from the human strain (*Entamoeba histolytica*).

Treatment is with metronidazole, with several dosages possible.
- 275 mg/kg via gastric tube, one dose (1)
- 125 mg/kg via gastric tube, one dose (1)
- Either dose given and then redosed q72–96 h prn (1)

Usually only one dose of either 125 mg/kg or 275 mg/kg is needed. In addition, give supportive treatment (e.g., fluids, force feeding) prn.

2. *Giardia* spp. *and Trichomonas* spp. (snakes, iguanas, turtles) are often seen on fecal examination. They must be differentiated from normal flora (*Nyctotherus*, *Balantidium*, and *Paramecium*). Treatment is with metronidazole (see the treatment listed for *Entamoeba invadens*).

3. Coccidial species seen include *Eimeria* (snakes, iguanas, turtles), *Isospora* (snakes, iguanas), and *Caryospora* (snakes, iguanas). They are seen asymptomatically or as a chronic gastrointestinal problem (especially in snakes). Treatment involves any of the sulfa drugs (see the description under *Cryptosporidium* spp.).

4. *Cryptosporidium* spp. (snakes, iguanas) can be transmitted from infected prey (especially mice). Signs in snakes include postprandial regurgitation and hypertrophic gastropathy (classically seen as a gross swelling of the stomach). In iguanas much less gastric hypertrophy is observed (possibly because the disease is more intestinal than gastric) (7). Usually, the animal is not anorectic but does show weight loss. Diagnosis is by gastric lavage and microscopic examination of the lavage fluid.

No effective treatment has been reported for *Cryptosporidium* spp. One report of treatment involved trimethoprim–sulfadiazine given orally at 60 mg/kg daily for 2 months; this snake was placed in a warmed environment (32 °C) and died

3 months after initial diagnosis. No necropsy was performed (1). In addition, treatment with 30–60 mg/kg PO, IM, SQ s.i.d. of trimethoprim–sulfadiazine can be tried (1,2). This disease is possibly zoonotic. The prey should ideally be screened for the presence of the organism.

Nematodes

Nematodes are commonly seen in many species of reptiles. The life cycles are usually direct, although intermediate hosts may be involved (*Ascaris* nematodes). Pets become infected by ingestion of ova or larvae and possibly by penetration of intact skin (*Strongylus* and *Trichostrongylus* nematodes). Symptoms depend upon the specific nematode and organ involved in the infestation. A parasitology text should be consulted for a more thorough discussion of these organisms.

■ PARASITES BY SPECIES OF PET

Iguanas

Common protozoa seen on a fecal flotation include *Entamoeba, Cryptosporidium, Trichomonas*, coccidia (*Eimeria, Isospora*, or *Caryospora*), and *Giardia*. Other parasites seen include *Oxyuris* spp. (pinworms) and *Strongyloides* spp.; many veterinarians consider all iguanas to have pinworms and deworm prophylactically (1). Often these parasites are diagnosed on an annual fecal examination from an otherwise asymptomatic animal.

Snakes

Common parasites include protozoal organisms such as *Entamoeba invadens, Eimeria, Isospora, Caryospora*, and *Cryptosporidium. Rhabditis, Strongyloides, Strongylus*, and *Trichostrongylus* nematodes are also encountered.

Turtles

Eimeria coccidia are seen as well as *Ascaris* and *Oxyuris*. While *Ascaris* can infect any reptile, turtles seem to be most commonly infected.

Treatment

Protozoa

1. Metronidazole: 40–125 mg/kg PO; repeat in 14 days.
2. Trimethoprim–Sulfadiazine: 30–60 mg/kg SQ, IM q24h for *Cryptosporidium*; use until cured (1,2).

Pinworms, Other Nematodes

1. Fenbendazole: 50–100 mg/kg PO; repeat in 14 days (1). Another regimen for turtles is to use 100 mg/kg by stomach tube q.o.d. for 3 days, and then repeat this process in 3 weeks.
2. Ivermectin: 0.2 mg/kg SQ, IM, PO; repeat in 14 days. *Do not use ivermectin in chelonians.*
3. Fenbendazole (Panacur 100 mg/mL) has been administered per-cloacally to tortoises infected with oxyurids. The tortoises were placed in dorsal recumbency and the tip of a lubricated TB syringe was gently inserted into the cloaca with manual pressure applied circumferentially around the cloaca to prevent leakage of medication. Expulsion of oxyurids occurred immediately and for 2–3 days after treatment; fecal flotations at 2 and 4 weeks after deworming failed to reveal ova. If possible, an attempt can be made to pass a red rubber catheter into the colon to prevent inadvertent passage of medication into the bladder. Per-cloacal administration of fenbendazole to tortoises or other species of reptiles may be an acceptable alternative to oral administration if this route is difficult or if several oral dewormings fail to eliminate the infection (8).

Coccidia

1. Sulfadiazine, sulfamerazine, sulfamethazine: 25 mg/kg s.i.d. for 10–14 days.
2. Trimethoprim–Sulfadiazine: 30 mg/kg SQ, IM, q24h for 10–14 days.

Note: Some parasites are difficult to eradicate with only two treatments. If ova are still seen after two treatments, continue for two more treatments, recheck the feces, and stop treatment once no more ova are detected.

Ivermectin *is fatal* when used in turtles and tortoises; another anthelmintic should be selected.

As a general rule, I use metronidazole (varying dosage) for protozoa, ivermectin (except in turtles) for nematodes, and trimethoprim–sulfa or Albon for coccidia.

■ **REFERENCES**

1.   Frye F. Reptile care: An atlas of diseases and treatments, vols. I and II. Neptune City, NJ: TFH, 1991.

2.   Jenkins J. Medical management of reptile patients. Compend Contin Educ Pract Vet, June 1991; 13:980–988.

3.   Raiti P. Veterinary care of the common kingsnake, *Lampropeltis getula*. Bull of ARAV 5:11–18.

4.   Anderson N. Husbandry and clinical evaluation of *Iguana iguana*. Compend Contin Educ Pract Vet, August 1991; 13:1265–1269.

5.   Mader, D. In Reptile Medicine and Surgery, WB Saunders, Philadelphia, PA, 1996:344

6.   Boyer T. Trichlorfon spray for snake mites (*Ophionyssus natricis*). Bull of ARAV, Premiere Issue, 1991:2.

7.   Boyer T. Common problems and treatment of green iguanas (*Iguana iguana*). Bull of ARAV, Premiere Issue, 1991:8–11.

8.   Innis C. Per-cloacal worming of tortoises. Bull of ARAV 5:4.

Appendices: Quick Reference Information

▼　　▼　　▼　　▼　　▼　　▼　　▼　　▼

Formulary

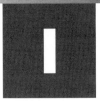

▼   ▼   ▼   ▼   ▼   ▼   ▼

A RRANGING a formulary creates some difficulty. Few if any drugs are approved for use in reptiles (or most pets for that matter). Much of what we know about pharmacology in reptiles is extrapolated from other species. Many of the drugs and dosages are derived from clinical experience rather than well-funded, basic research. There are many "formularies" available, each of which seems to have different drugs and dosages. The following is the formulary I use in practice. There are more drugs available to the practitioner, but since this book deals mainly with common diseases of iguanas, snakes, and turtles, I have tried to include only the drugs and dosages commonly used in these pets. As is true with so many formularies, a disclaimer is necessary. You are advised to warn owners of the off-label use of drugs in treating their reptiles; some veterinarians have owners sign release forms.

While multiple forms and dosages often exist for a drug, it is ultimately up to the individual practitioner to make an appropriate selection for treatment based upon the species of pet, its size, its age, the presence of concurrent problems, contraindications of the drug, cost of the medication, ease of administration, and preference based upon clinical experience.

■ ANTIBIOTICS

Amikacin sulfate: 2.5 mg/kg SQ, IM every 72 hours for 5–7 treatments. 1.0 mg/kg in the blood python *Python curtis*; 2.0 mg/kg in the black-headed python *Aspidites melanocephalus* and rock python *Liasis macloti*. Some authors have suggested an initial dose of 2.5 mg/kg, followed by 1.5 mg/kg in blood pythons. Is often combined with a beta-lactam antibiotic, such as piperacillin, or a cephalosporin. Less nephrotoxic than gentamicin or tobramycin. Many authors recommend fluid therapy whenever aminoglycosides are given,* although I have not experienced renal toxicity in animals that were active, eating and drinking, and not receiving supplemental fluids. Can be used for nebulization at 2 mg/10 mL saline prn (1,2).

Carbenicillin: 400 mg/kg IM s.i.d. (3).

Cefotaxime: 20–40 mg/kg IM s.i.d. (1).

Cephalothin: 40–80 mg/kg IM dd b.i.d. (1).

Cephaloridine: 10 mg/kg IM, SQ b.i.d. Maintain hydration (1).

Chloramphenicol succinate: 20 mg/kg SQ, IM b.i.d. Useful for some anaerobic infections (2).

Doxycycline: 5–10 mg/kg PO s.i.d. for 10–45 days. Useful for some anaerobic infections. Probably should combine with nystatin during prolonged use to prevent secondary yeast infections (2).

Enrofloxacin: 10 mg/kg SQ, IM q24h for 10–14 days. May cause skin discoloration or tissue necrosis if given SQ. May be used as a nasal flush (50 mg/250 mL of sterile water or saline) by giving 1–3 mL/nostril s.i.d. (2,4). An alternative dose is 2.5–5.0 mg/kg PO, IM b.i.d. (1). For box turtles, a dosage of 5 mg/kg IM q96–120h is recommended (3).

Piperacillin: 200–400 mg/kg IM q24h. Some authors advocate 100 mg/kg q48h in blood pythons (3). Excellent broad-spectrum antibiotic. Should be combined with amikacin. Use the lower dose in combination with amikacin. Some authors advocate fluid therapy when using piperacillin, especially in combination with amikacin (2). An alternative dose is 50–100 mg/kg IM s.i.d. (1). I have used it alone and in combination with amikacin. When cost is a factor (larger pets), I will use 400 mg/kg as a loading dose for 2–3 days and then 100–200 mg/kg for maintenance.

Tetracycline/Oxytetracycline: 10 mg/kg PO s.i.d. Useful for some anaerobic infections (1). Combine with nystatin during prolonged use to prevent secondary yeast infections.

---

* Some veterinarians advise parenteral fluids whenever an aminoglycoside is used. Bacterial diseases should be treated for a minimum of 2–3 weeks; anaerobic culturing is often recommended at the beginning of treatment or if no response is seen in 2–3 weeks.

Trimethoprim–Sulfadiazine: 30 mg/kg SQ, IM q24h for 10–14 treatments. Is safe, and can be used to treat coccidiosis. Coccidiosis can also be treated with an oral sulfadiazine dose of 25 mg/kg (2). An alternative dose is 15–30 mg/kg SQ, IM s.i.d. (1,4).

■ **TOPICAL ANTIBIOTICS**

Chlorhexidine diacetate solution: 0.25–1.0% solution, prn (1).

Povidone–iodine solution: 0.5–1.0% solution, prn (1).

Silvadene: As needed. Good for burns and infectious stomatitis (1).

Acetic acid (vinegar): Can use straight or as a 0.5% solution. Used for infectious stomatitis (1).

Dakin's solution (sodium hypochlorite, bleach): Available as a 5.25% stock solution. Dilute to 0.5% solution (1).

Preparation H: Can be used to reduce edema associated with a prolapsed cloaca or hemipenes prior to surgical replacement (5).

Betadine, Panalog, and Furacin ointments can also be used as topical antibiotics in reptiles (1).

■ **ANTIFUNGALS**

Amphotericin B: 1.0 mg/kg diluted with water or saline intratracheally q24h for 2–4 weeks. Used for treating fungal pneumonia (2).

Ketoconazole: 50.0 mg/kg PO b.i.d. for 2–4 weeks. Used for deep fungal and yeast infections (12). In turtles, the recommended dosage is 15 mg/kg q24h given in food (2).

Nystatin: 100,000 IU/kg PO q24h. Used for gastrointestinal yeast infections (2,3).

■ **PARASITICIDES**

External Parasites

Dichlorvos strip: Hung within 6 in. of the cage (not in it) for 3 days; remove for 7 days; repeat regimen four times (5).

Ivermectin: 0.2 mg/kg SQ, IM, PO; repeat in 10–14 days. *Contraindicated in animals who have or will be treated with diazepam within 10 days, and in turtles and tortoises.* May cause skin discoloration if given SQ (1,2).

Pyrethrin kitten spray: First spray only the cage once; 3 days later, spray the cage and tail; if no signs of toxicity are noted, spray *lightly* the entire cage and lizard or snake every 3 days for 3 weeks. Can also spray a cloth and then rub the pet with the cloth (5). Mader has used Durakyl (Dum Pharmaceuticals, Miami, FL) which contains 0.35% Resmethrin, effectively and safely in treating reptiles with mite infestations (6).

Snake mites have been successfully treated using Permectrin spray (Permectrin II, Bio-Ceutic). The stock compound was diluted to a 1% solution with tap water and applied to snakes using a spray bottle. After disinfecting the cage, bowls, and hiding boxes with Roccal-D (Winthrop Laboratories), the cage and water bowls and hiding boxes were thoroughly sprayed; excess spray was removed with paper towel. The snake was lightly sprayed, excess spray wiped with a paper towel, and the snake placed in a clean holding cage for 24 hours. The procedure was repeated in 10 days, and again in 10 days if a third treatment was needed. The snake should be washed with water 1 day prior to treatment.

Only one toxic reaction was seen in a snake treated 10 days earlier with 2% Trichlorfon solution. The snake, which exhibited convulsions, ataxia, and open-mouth breathing, was treated with fluids and corticosteroids. Complete recovery occurred within 5 days (7).

I have observed one toxic reaction in a small infant kingsnake that was sprayed with pyrethrin flea spray (approved for cats). The snake exhibited tremors and bizarre behavior immediately after being sprayed. The spray was immediately removed with careful rinsing of the snake with soap and water; one injection of diazepam was given IM. The snake was placed in a dark cage; the behavior lessened but was still present. The behavior was worse if the room lights were turned on and the snake was handled (i.e., worse signs appeared when the snake was stimulated). No other treatment was instituted, and the snake recovered within 24 hours.

Pyrethrin-type sprays should be used cautiously in snakes and other reptiles; pyrethroid sprays may be safer than Pyrethrin products.

Sevin Dust (5% carbaryl): For treating snake mites. Remove the snake from the cage. Wash the cage and its furnishings with soap and water, rinse, wash with 5% bleach, rinse, and dry thoroughly. Sprinkle Sevin Dust in the cage. Return only the snake to the cage for 24 hours. Remove it, clean and dry the cage, wipe excess dust off of the snake, and then return the snake and the furnishings to the cage. Repeat in 2 weeks.

Another successful protocol with carbaryl dust involves dusting the snake and leaving the powder on for 30 minutes. The snake is then washed with tap water. The cage must also be disinfected (6).

Trichlorfon spray (Trichlorfon pour-on cattle insecticide, Chem-Tronics, Inc., Leavenworth, Kansas) diluted to 0.15% (8 mL of stock 8% solution with 400 mL of water): Clean the cage and furnishings with 3% bleach, dry them, add newspaper as the substrate, and then lightly spray this set-up with the 0.15% Trichlorfon and allow it to dry *before* replacing the reptile. The reptile is *lightly* sprayed, and water is withheld for 24 hours so the pet doesn't accidentally soak and ingest the Trichlorfon. Repeat in 2 weeks. The diluted solution remains stable for about 1 month (8).

Internal Parasites

Protozoa (Amoeba, Trichomonads)

Metronidazole: 40–125 mg/kg PO; repeat in 14 days. Lower dosages are used in tricolor kingsnakes and indigo snakes. A dosage interval of q72h for 5–7 doses is recommended for treating *Entamoeba invadens* (2). Frye recommends 50–125 mg PO via stomach tube once to help stimulate appetite in anorectic snakes (1).

Cryptosporidia

Trimethoprim–Sulfadiazine: 30 mg/kg PO, SQ, IM q24h; use until cured (2). An alternative dose is 60 mg/kg PO s.i.d. for 2 months or longer (1).

Pinworms, Other Nematodes

Fenbendazole (Panacur): 50–100 mg/kg PO; repeat in 14 days (1). In turtles with nematodes, use 100 mg/kg PO OD for three treatments. Repeat in 2–3 weeks, and check a fecal sample in 1–2 months. Retreat prn. Fenbendazole powder can be mixed with the food (for larger pets) or given as a slurry via a stomach tube (8).

Ivermectin: 0.2 mg/kg SQ, IM, PO; repeat in 14 days. Is *lethal* to, and should be avoided in turtles and tortoises. There are reports of discolored skin in (colored) reptiles given the medication SQ. *Con-*

traindicated in animals who have been, or will be, treated with diazepam within 10 days (1,2).

Coccidia

Sulfadiazine, sulfamerazine, sulfamethazine: 25 mg/kg s.i.d. for 10–14 days (2). Another protocol recommends 75 mg/kg on day 1, then 40 mg/kg for the next 5 days (9).

Sulfadimethoxine (Albon): 90 mg/kg day 1, 45 mg/kg 5 days (10).

Trimethoprim–Sulfadiazine: 30 mg/kg SQ, IM q24h for 10–14 days (10).

Cestodes/Trematodes

Praziquantel: 8–20 mg/kg PO, IM; repeat in 14 days (2).

Note: Some parasites, specifically nematodes, are difficult to eradicate with only two treatments. If ova are still seen after two treatments, continue for two more treatments, recheck the stool, and stop treatment once no more ova are detected.

■ ANESTHETICS

General, Inhalants

Aerrane: Anesthetic of choice. The reptile can be induced by box or mask, or by an injectable anesthetic and then maintained on Aerrane.

General, Injectable

Ketamine: 20–60 mg/kg IM, SQ (see "Anesthesia" in chapter 5 for dosage by species and precautions). Induction occurs within 5 minutes; arousal occurs within 45 minutes. Can use diazepam if seizures or tonic–clonic movements are seen (rare). *Contraindicated in renal disease.* Can be reversed with Yohimbine. Elimination can be increased with fluids and diuretics. Use lower dose for shorter procedures (1,2).

Telazol: 10–30 mg/kg IM (see "Anesthesia" in chapter 5 for dosage by species). Same comments as with ketamine, although diazepam should not be needed as zolazepam is included in Telazol. *Contraindicated if ivermectin has been used, or will be used, within 10 days due to zolazepam fraction.* Use lower dose for shorter procedures (1).

An alternative dose is 20–40 mg/kg for iguanas and snakes, 5–15 mg/kg for turtles (2).

Immobilization (see Anesthesia)

Succinylcholine: 0.25–1.0 mg/kg IM. An effect is seen within 20–60 minutes; it lasts 1–4 hours. Used for short-term restraint in chelonians to allow the head and limbs to be withdrawn from the shell. If higher dosages are used, respiration may need to be assisted. Occasionally, a chelonian will rigidly extend its limbs for 1–2 minutes after the injection; respiration should be monitored and assisted if needed. Succinylcholine provides no anesthesia or analgesia (2).

Local (1–2% Lidocaine): Rarely used. Can be used for minor procedures (e.g., suturing) and may need to be combined with sedation. Use the lowest possible dose needed.

Hypothermia: Used in the past for immobilization/anesthesia. Hypothermia, while it can immobilize reptiles and decrease their metabolism, is *not* an anesthetic or analgesic and should not be used for these purposes. By decreasing metabolic rate, hypothermia can diminish an animal's immune response to disease. Hypothermia should be abandoned for use in reptiles.

Analeptics: Dopram (20 mg/mL), 0.25 mL/kg IV (11).

Anticholinergics

Atropine: 0.01–0.04 mg/kg IM, IV for premedication (1); 0.1–0.2 mg/kg for organophosphate toxicity (2); 0.04–0.1 mg/kg for bradycardia (2). Also used in infectious stomatitis (s.i.d.–t.i.d.) at 0.04 mg/kg PO, IV, IM, SQ to dry up oral secretions.

Glycopyrolate: 10 μg/kg SQ, IM, IV. Same indication as in mammals. Could possibly substitute for atropine in the treatment of infectious stomatitis (1).

■ MISCELLANEOUS

Allopurinol: Can be tried for gout by mixing one 100 mg tablet (crushed) in 10 mL of water and giving 1 drop/30 g PO q.i.d. (11). A dosage of 20 mg/kg PO s.i.d. in turtles and kingsnakes has been reported (13).

Arginine vasotocin: 0.01–1.0 μm/kg IV, IP prn for dystocia.

Administer 0.2–0.5 mL/kg of Calphosan IM, SQ prior to arginine vasotocin. Many practitioners feel arginine vasotocin is more efficacious in treating dystocia in reptiles than oxytocin (5,13).

Butorphanol (Torbugesic, Torbutrol): 0.5–1.0 mg/kg IM postoperatively in chelonians for pain due to shell fractures.

Calcium gluconate 10%: (100 mg/mL), 500 mg/kg intracoelemically weekly for 4–6 weeks for treatment of metabolic bone disease (1,14). Dosage of 10–50 mg/kg IM when used for dystocia (2).

Calcium glycerophosphate and lactate (Calphosan): 0.5–1.0 mL/kg (50–100 mg/kg) IM weekly for 4–6 weeks for metabolic bone disease (5). Dosage of 1.0–2.5 mL/kg (100–250 mg/kg) given prior to oxytocin for dystocia (2). Dosage of 0.2–0.5 mL/kg (20–50 mg/kg) given prior to arginine vasotocin for dystocia (5).

Calcitonin (Calcimar): Supplied as a stock solution of 200 IU/mL that is diluted with sterile PSS to a final strength of 1.0 IU/mL and dosed at 1.5 units/kg SQ t.i.d. Used to treat hypervitaminosis D (hypercalcemia) (1).

For the treatment of metabolic bone disease in iguanas, a dose of 50 IU/kg IM (15). Supplement with Neo-Calglucon at 1 mL/kg (23 mg/kg) PO b.i.d. if blood calcium levels are normal, decreased, or not known (see "Metabolic Bone Disease" in chapter 6).

Dexamethasone: 0.0625–0.125 mg/kg IV, IM for shock (1).

Dexamethasone sodium phosphate: 0.10–0.25 mg/kg IV, IM for septic shock (2).

Emeraid II: 10–15 ml/500 g SID–BID of product after rehydration (dilute 1:1 to 1:6 with warm water).

Fluids (lactated Ringer's, PSS): 15–25 mL/kg/day for maintenance ICe, ECe, SC (ICe: intracoelomic; ECe: epicoelomic, SC: subcutaneous). Fluids are given either intracoelomically or epico-elomically. As a rule, the dosage corresponds to 1–3% of the pet's body weight (1).

Two formulas are available for making a "Reptile Ringer's solution," which may be more physiologically correct than LRS as a replacement fluid for reptiles (10):

- Mix 1 part plain Ringer's with 2 parts 2.5% dextrose and 0.45% saline.
- Mix 1 part D5W with 1 part 0.9% saline and 1 part LRS.

Furosemide: 5 mg/kg IV, IM prn. Useful for reducing respiratory fluid volume in severe respiratory diseases. Can also be used in situations analogous to mammals (e.g., edema, heart failure). When diuretics are used, parenteral fluids are usually indicated to prevent volume depletion (1).

Methimazole: 1.0–1.25 mg/kg PO s.i.d. for 30 days for hyperthyroidism in snakes. Determine the thyroid value before and during treatment. Adjust dosage to lowest possible dose after 4 months of treatment. May need lifelong therapy (1).

Neo-Calglucon: 1 mL/kg (23 mg/kg) PO b.i.d. prn when used with calcitonin for treating metabolic bone disease in iguanas (15).

Oxytocin: 1–10 IU/kg IM. Usually used in conjunction with calcium for dystocia. Many doctors prefer arginine vasotocin and question the efficacy of oxytocin when used to treat dystocia in reptiles (2, 5).

Prednisolone: 0.50–1.0 mg/kg IM, SQ, PO s.i.d. (for immunosuppression, avian dosage) (12).

Propylthiouracil: 10 mg/kg PO s.i.d. for 21–30 days for hyperthyroidism in snakes. Determine the thyroid value before and during treatment. Adjust dosage to lowest possible dose after 4 months of treatment. May need lifelong therapy (1).

Vitamins A, D, and E: Several dosages are used:

- 0.15 mL/kg IM, repeated in 21 days for hypovitaminosis A and hypovitaminosis D_3 (2).
- In turtles with hypovitaminosis A, 0.1 mL Injacom-100 (Roche)/300 g PO initial dose, then 0.02 mL/week for 2–3 more weeks PO.
- 2000 IU/kg Aquasol A parenteral (Armour) SQ once weekly for 4–6 weeks. At 2000 IU/kg, this regimen is usually 0.01–0.02 mL/week.

Injacom A has too much vitamin A per mL to give parenterally as hypervitaminosis A may result (hypervitaminosis A has resulted when vitamin A was given parenterally at 5000 IU/kg) (1, 4). For metabolic bone disease in iguanas, dose Injacom-100 at 100 IU of vitamin D_3/kg SQ with two total doses; each dose is given 1 week apart (14).

B-complex vitamins: 0.25–0.50 mL/kg IM. Empirical dosage (2).

Vitamin C: Dosage is empirical, and two doses have been reported: 10–20 mg/kg IM s.i.d. (1) and 100–250 mg/kg IM s.i.d. (2). Used by some veterinarians when treating infectious stomatitis or severe burns.

Vitamin K: 0.25–0.75 mg/kg IM. Useful for suspected vitamin K deficient clotting problems (1).

■ REFERENCES

1. Frye F. Reptile care: An atlas of diseases and treatments, vols. I and II. Neptune City, NJ: TFH, 1991.

2. Jenkins J. Medical management of reptile patients. Compend Contin Educ Pract Vet, June 1991; 13:980–988.

3. Jacobson ER. Antimicrobial drug use in reptiles. In: Prescott JF, Baggot JD. Antimicrobial therapy in veterinary medicine, 2nd ed. Ames: Iowa State University Press, 1993:52.

4. Boyer T. Common problems of box turtles (*Terrapene* spp.) in captivity. Bull of ARAV 2:9–16.

5. Anderson N. Husbandry and clinical evaluation of *Iguana iguana*. Compend Contin Educ Pract Vet, August 1991; 13:1265–1269.

6. Mader, D. In Peptile Medicine and Surgery, WB Saunders, Philadelphia, PA; 1996; 344.

7. Boyer D. Snake mite (*Ophionyssus natricis*) eradication utilizing Permectrin spray. Bull of ARAV 5:4–5.

8. Boyer T, Boyer D. Trichlorfon spray for snake mites (*Ophionyssus natricis*). Bull of ARAV, 1991; Premiere Issue:2–3.

9. Funk RS. Herp health hints and husbandry: Parasiticide dosages for captive amphibians and reptiles. Bull Chicago Herp Soc, 1988; 23:30.

10. Monograph formulary. In: Bull of ARAV 5:27–28.

11. Boyer T. Clinical anesthesia of reptiles. Bull of ARAV 2:10–12.

12. Ritchie B, *et al.* Avian medicine: Principles and applications. Lake Worth: Wingers, 1994:458.

13. Raiti P. Veterinary care of the common kingsnake, *Lampropeltis getula*. Bull of ARAV 5:11–18.

14. Boyer T. Common problems and treatment of the green iguana (*Iguana iguana*). Bull of ARAV, Premiere Issue:8–11.

15. Mader D. Use of calcitonin in green iguanas, *Iguana iguana*, with metabolic bone disease. Bull of ARAV 3:5.

Common Supplies

1/2 mL TB syringes with 27- or 28-gauge needles

Feeding tubes

Plastic tom cat urinary catheters

Sexing probes

Plastic spatulas

Incubator

Gram scale

Surgical instruments (Iris scissors, small hemostats, tissue forceps, jeweler's forceps, small scissors, and needle holders)

Fine suture material (3-0–6-0 Vicryl/PDS)

Operating microscope/OptiVisor

Iguana Diet

■ OPTION I

THERE IS controversy surrounding what is the "best" diet to feed an iguana. Previously, it was recommended to feed based on the "life-stage" of the pet, with the younger iguanas receiving a larger amount of animal-based protein and the older iguanas receiving less animal-based protein (Option I). Some veterinarians are currently recommending a diet that is 100% plant-based with no animal protein in the diet (option II). Their recommendation is based on research that showed that the stomach contents of iguanas (in the wild) consisted entirely of plant material with no evidence of animal protein such as insects, arachnids, or eggs. It is up to each veterinarian to decide which diet he or she prefers to recommend to clients. As long as the amount of animal-based protein is a small part of the diet, I currently recommend Option I. If the iguana refuses to eat animal-based material, that is also acceptable.

For juvenile iguanas, 80% of the diet should be plant-based protein material and 20% animal-based protein material. For adult iguanas, 90% of the diet should be plant-based and 10% animal-based (alternatively, adult iguanas can be fed 100% vegetable material). Of the plant matter, most (80%) should be vegetable- or flower-based, and only 20% fruit-based.

Acceptable plant-based matter:

Alfalfa chow or hay
Bell pepper
Bok choy
Broccoli
Cabbage

Cactus
Collard/mustard/turnip greens
Corn
Flowers: carnations, hibiscus, roses (azaleas are toxic and should be avoided)
Green beans
Green peas
Kale
Okra
Parsley
Spinach (less than 10% of the vegetable matter, as spinach contains oxalates that bind calcium)
Sweet potatoes
Yellow squash/zucchini/acorn squash
Fruit:
Apples
Bananas
Figs
Grapes
Peaches
Kiwi
Melons
Papayas
Pears
Raspberries
Strawberries

Appropriate animal-based protein sources include crickets, sardines (drained), tofu, hard-boiled eggs, earthworms, and mealworms. Dog food and cat food contain too much vitamin D and fat and should be avoided. Reptile pellets, bird pellets, trout chow, and other fish chows are excellent animal-based protein sources; feeding these items precludes the need for live prey.

■ OPTION II

All iguanas regardless of age should be fed a diet of only plant-based material Acceptable items are mentioned in Option I.

Calcium Content of Common Foods

▼   ▼   ▼   ▼   ▼   ▼   ▼   ▼

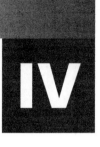

	(100-g Sample)
Apple	6.0 mg
Green beans	56 mg
Broccoli	88 mg
Carrot tops	310 mg
Alfalfa (dry)	1700 mg
Potato	5 mg
Iceburg lettuce	19 mg
Celery	20 mg
Squash (many varieties)	28 mg
Sweet potato	29 mg
Lima beans	52 mg
Romaine lettuce	67 mg
Spinach	93 mg
Fescue grass	130 mg
Dandelion greens	187 mg
Collard greens	203 mg
Parsley	203 mg
Kale	249 mg
Turnip greens	246 mg
Opuntia cactus	1890 mg

Adapted from Atlas of Nutritional Data of United States and Canadian Feeds, National Academy of Science, Washington, D.C., 1971; and Adams, C.F., Agricultural handbook #456 Nutritive Value of American Foods in Common Units, 1975.

Treatment Protocol for
Metabolic Bone Disease

▼　▼　▼　▼　▼　▼　▼　▼

V

■ OPTION I

1. 10% calcium gluconate, (100 mg/mL), 500 mg/kg intracoelomically weekly for 4–6 weeks; or Calphosan 0.5–1.0 mL/kg IM
weekly for 4–6 weeks; or Neo-Calglucon at 1 mL/kg (23 mg/
kg) b.i.d. PO for 2–3 months while diet is corrected.
2. B-complex vitamin injection: 0.25–0.50 mL/kg, once.
3. Injacom-100: Dose at 100 IU vitamin D_3/kg SQ, two doses 1
week apart.

■ OPTION II

1. Start calcium glubionate (Neo-Calglucon syrup, USP) at
1 mL/kg (23 mg/kg) PO q12h on the first visit. Calcium gluconate (100 mg/kg IM or ICe q6h prn for up to 24 hours) can
be given if hypocalcemic tetany is present. After stabilization
(usually 2–3 months), you may switch to an s.i.d. regimen.
2. Injacom-100 (dosed at 1000 IU vitamin D_3/kg) IM once weekly
for two treatments at week 1 and week 2 visits.
3. Calcitonin (Calcimar, 200 IU/mL) at 50 IU/kg IM once weekly
at the week 2 and 3 visits.

Severely ill iguanas should be hospitalized for intensive care;
appropriate laboratory tests should be run to check for concurrent
problems.

Sources: Option 1: Boyer T. Common Problems and Treatment of
Green Iguanas (*Iguana iguana*). AARV Premiere Issue, 1991:8–11.
Option II: Boyer T. Metabolic Bone Disease. In Reptile Medicine and
Surgery. Mader, D. WB Saunders, Phil, PA 1996:385–392.

Treatment Protocol for Infectious Stomatitis

▼ ▼ ▼ ▼ ▼ ▼ ▼ ▼

■ **MILD CASES**

1. Culture and sensitivity test of the oral cavity (possibly including anaerobic cultures).
2. Begin therapy with any of the following antibiotics, pending C&S results: (see Formulary for an in-depth discussion).
   - Amikacin: 2.5 mg/kg SQ, IM every 72 hours for 5–7 treatments
   - Piperacillin: 200–400 mg/kg IM q24h
   - Cephalothin: 40–80 mg/kg dd b.i.d.
   - Trimethoprim–Sulfadiazine: 30 mg/kg SQ, IM q24h for 10–14 treatments
3. Oral therapy to include any of the following topical rinses:
   - Dilute chlorhexidine solution (0.25–0.50%)
   - Dilute povidone–iodine solution (1%)
   - Acetic acid (vinegar) (dilute to a 0.5% solution)
   - Hydrogen peroxide

   Rinses are given b.i.d.; the mouth is rinsed with plain water after the rinses are used. Alternating rinses (i.e., chlorhexidine day 1, peroxide day 2, acetic acid day 3, with the pattern then repeated for the duration of treatment) may be helpful. I alternate rinses as follows: chlorhexidine followed by peroxide followed by tap water on day 1, chlorhexidine followed by vinegar followed by water on day 2, and with this regimen repeated on subsequent days. The vinegar (acetic acid) produces an acid environment; the peroxide produces an oxygenated environment that is not conducive to anaerobic organisms. Wear eye protection (goggles) and have clients do the same when rinsing the oral cavity!

4. Topical Silvadene applied after oral rinses.

■ **SEVERE CASES**

1. In addition to the treatment listed for mild cases, severely ill pets need hospitalization with fluid therapy (15–25 mL/kg/day for maintenance), incubation (85–95 °F), and force feeding.

2. In addition, you may want to use enrofloxacin +/− amikacin as your initial antibiotic selection.

    • Enrofloxacin: 10 mg/kg IM q24h for 10–14 days

The use of parenteral fluids in any reptile receiving aminoglycosides should be strongly considered to prevent renal damage.

For cases that don't respond to appropriate antimicrobial therapy, consider an anaerobic infection. Perform an anaerobic culture and treat with metronidazole, clindamycin, or tetracycline. Anaerobes may account for as much as 50% of bacterial infections in reptiles.

Treatment Protocol for Hypovitaminosis A

▼ ▼ ▼ ▼ ▼ ▼ ▼ ▼

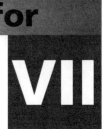

1. 0.1 mL Injacom-100 (Roche, 100,000 IU vitamin A/mL)/300 g PO initial dose, then 0.02 mL/week for 2–3 more weeks PO; or 2000 IU/kg Aquasol A parenteral (Armour) SQ once weekly for 4–6 weeks. At 2000 IU/kg, this regimen is usually 0.01–0.02 mL/week. Injacom-100 has too much vitamin A per mL to give parenterally, as hypervitaminosis A may result.
2. Slowly improve the diet and have the owner begin using reptile or avian vitamins.
3. Treat secondary problems.

Source: Boyer T. Common Problems of Box Turtles (*Terrapene sppl* in captivity, AARV vol 2, No 1:9–14.

Fluid Therapy Guide

▼ ▼ ▼ ▼ ▼ ▼ ▼ ▼

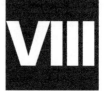

VIII

LACTATED Ringer's/Physiologic Saline Solution (PSS): 15–25 mL/kg/day ICe, ECe, SC (ICe: intracoelomic; ECe: epicoelomic; SC: subcutaneous). As a rule, the dosage corresponds to 1–3% of the pet's body weight. Warming the fluid may be beneficial.

Two formulas are available for making a "Reptile Ringer's solution," which may be more physiologically correct than lactated Ringer's solution as a replacement fluid for reptiles:

- Mix 1 part plain Ringer's with 2 parts 2.5% dextrose and 0.45% saline.
- Mix 1 part D5W with 1 part 0.9% saline and 1 part lactated Ringer's solution (LRS) or PSS.

■ REHYDRATION

Water Soaks

Turtles and tortoises (and possibly other reptiles) can absorb water through their cloacal openings. All hospitalized reptiles can benefit from several (t.i.d.) 5- to 15-minute soaks in warm water (80–90 °F), in addition to injectable rehydration therapy. *Care must be taken to ensure that the animal does not drown in the water bath.*

Intracoelomic Injections

The intracoelomic (turtles, snakes, and iguanas), epicoelomic (turtles), and subcutaneous routes are used for fluid therapy. In making injections, advance the needle just far enough to enter the coelomic cavity without penetrating viscera. Needle lengths and gauges vary according to the size of the pet. For most small iguanas and turtles, as well as most snakes of any size, a 1-in., 22–25 gauge needle suffices.

For iguanas: Inject into the caudal paralumbar abdominal space, which is located in front of the femur about one-third the distance ventrally from the dorsal midline. The animal struggles less if the injection is given in this location while it is in a normal "sitting" posture. Injections can be given in the caudal ventral abdomen with the iguana placed on its back; the iguana seems to struggle more in this position, however. Subcutaneous injections are given in the dorsal flank, axillary, or interscapular area.

For snakes: An injection is made anywhere along the ventrum of the snake. Ideally, the needle passes between, and not through, the scales. Insert the needle only enough to penetrate the coelomic membrane and enter the body cavity. Alternatively, SQ fluids can be given in the lateral sinus, which is located at the junction between the epaxial muscles and the ribs.

For turtles: Intracoelomic injections are made just cranial to the hindlimb. An epicoelomic injection is approached by directing the needle caudally just ventral to the shoulder joint (pectoral girdle) and dorsal to the plastron; the needle is passed through the pectoral muscles into the epicoelomic space, and directed toward the contralateral hindlimb. Epicoelomic injections are preferred if the turtle is suffering from severe respiratory disease (pneumonia). Epicoelomic injections also avoid possible lung laceration (which may occur with intracoelomic injections) and do not compromise lung space within the shell cavity.

Force-Feeding Guide

▼   ▼   ▼   ▼   ▼   ▼   ▼   ▼

IX

STOMACH volume is estimated at 2% of body weight, or 20 mL/ kg.

For snakes: The stomach is located at the junction of the second and third quarters of the snake's body. If possible, pass the tube into the stomach. Otherwise, in longer snakes, the tube is passed into the esophagus.

For iguanas: Measure the distance from the nose to the last rib. Open the mouth, and note and avoid the trachea. An appropriate speculum can be used to hold the mouth open (e.g., a plastic syringe case). The feeding tube is passed the premeasured distance through the esophagus into the stomach. Alternatively, in small iguanas (less than 100 g), a 1 mL TB syringe without a needle can be used for the feeding. The syringe is passed through the esophagus into the stomach while slowly twirling the syringe. It is passed one-third of the distance from the front legs to the rear legs to arrive in the stomach.

For turtles: Gently extend the neck and hold the turtle vertically. Measure the distance from the center of the plastron (where the stomach lies) to the front of the maxilla with the neck extended. Gently open the mouth and insert a speculum (a paper clip is used for small turtles; small mouth specula or hemostats also work). Pass the lubricated tube down the esophagus and into the stomach. Avoid the glottis at the base of the tongue. Keep the turtle vertical for 1 minute after feeding. Some box turtles and iguanas will eat without tube feeding if the food is placed into the oral cavity with a syringe.

Consider an esophagostomy tube if repeated force feedings are necessary and if the animal is easily stressed.

■ DIETS

For iguanas and box turtles: Use 1 part Emeraid II diluted with 1–3 parts warm water. The mixture should be made fresh at each feeding. The empirical dosage is 2.5 mL/100 g s.i.d.–t.i.d. Another option is to mix 1 part alfalfa pellets with 2 parts warm water, and feed this mixture at 20 mL/kg q.o.d. for iguanas with a body weight of more than 50 g. Make sure pets are adequately hydrated (through the use of oral or intracoelomic fluid administration) prior to force feeding.

For snakes: Mix Emeraid II and 1–3 parts warm water and enough turkey baby food to make a slurry. This mixture is fed at a dosage of 10–20 mL/ft of snake (2.5–5.0 mL/100 g, or approximately 10–20 mL/1b). Feed at least as often as the snake normally eats (usually every 1–4 weeks), sometimes more often. Another acceptable diet is a slurry made with beaten raw eggs and meat-based baby food, fed in the same amounts as mentioned above. It is important that snakes not be handled if at all possible for at least 48–72 hours post-prandially; vomiting may result, and complete digestion takes 3–4 days. Treatments that need to be given post-prandially should be performed quickly and with minimal stress to the patient.

Normal Blood Values for Boas and Pythons

▼   ▼   ▼   ▼   ▼   ▼   ▼   ▼

	Boa	*Python*
WBC ($\times 10^3$/mm^3)	4–10	6–12
RBC ($\times 10^6$/mm^3)	1.0–2.5	1.0–2.5
PCV (%)	24–40	25–40
Bands (%)	0	0
Neutrophils (%)	0–15	0–15
Heterophils (%)	20–50	20–60
Lymphocytes (%)	10–60	10–60
Monocytes (%)	0–3	0–3
Eosinophils (%)	0–3	0–3
Basophils (%)	0–20	0–10
SGOT/AST (IU/L)	5–35	5–30
Total protein (g/dL)	4.6–8.0	5.0–8.0
LDH (IU/L)	30–300	40–300
Calcium (mg/dL)	10–22	10–22
Glucose (mg/dL)	10–60	10–60
Uric acid (mg/dL)	1.2–5.8	1.2–5.6
Potassium (mEq/L)	3.0–5.7	3.0–5.7
Sodium (mEq/L)	130–152	130–152

Source: Rosskopf WJ, Woerpel RW, Yanoff SR. Normal hemogram and blood chemistry values for boa constrictors and pythons. VM/SAC, May 1982:822–823.

Normal Blood Values for the California Desert Tortoise

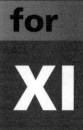

▼ ▼ ▼ ▼ ▼ ▼ ▼ ▼

WBC ($\times 10^3/\text{mm}^3$)	3.1–9.3
RBC ($\times 10^6/\text{mm}^3$)	0.5–0.9
PCV (%)	25–53
Neutrophils (%)	0–1
Heterophils (%)	46–81
Lymphocytes (%)	3–23
Monocytes (%)	0–2
Eosinophils (%)	0–1
Basophils (%)	0–39
SGOT/AST (IU/L)	0–118
Total protein (g/dL)	2.3–5.0
Albumin (g/dL)	0.7–1.9
Calcium (mg/dL)	4.8–16.7
Phosphorus (mg/dL)	1.2–4.4
Glucose (mg/dL)	40–91
Uric acid (mg/dL)	0–4
Potassium (mEq/L)	2.7–6.0
Sodium (mEq/L)	128–149
T_3 (ng/dL)	11–72
T_4 (µg/dL)	0–1.0
Free T_4 (ng/dL)	0–0.7

Source: Clinical laboratory normals: California desert tortoise. PAL News, Winter 1992–1993:7.

▼

Normal Blood Values for the Green Iguana

WBC ($\times 10^3/mm^3$)	4.3–15.0
RBC ($\times 10^6/mm^3$)	3.5–5.8
PCV (%)	45–52
Heterophils (%)	5–55
Lymphocytes (%)	35–55
Monocytes (%)	<4%
Eosinophils (%)	<2%
Basophils (%)	rare
SGOT/AST (IU/L)	6–168
Total protein (g/dL)	4.3–7.3
Calcium (mg/dL)	9.7–14.1
Phosphorus (mg/dL)	4.7–9.3
Glucose (mg/dL)	120–286
Uric acid (mg/dL)	1.3–5.3
Potassium (mEq/L)	1.8–3.8
Sodium (mEq/L)	152–164

Sources: Anderson N. Diseases of *Iguana iguana*. Compend Contin Educ Pract Vet, Oct 1992; 14:1335–1342 (hematology); and Southwest Veterinary Diagnostic Laboratories, normal blood values (biochemistries).

Interpretation of the Blood Profile

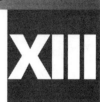

▼   ▼   ▼   ▼   ▼   ▼   ▼   ▼

XIII

PROTEIN: 3–8 g/dL normal range.

Hypoproteinemia is seen with malnutrition, malabsorption, maldigestion, intestinal parasitism, severe blood loss, chronic renal disease, chronic hepatic disease, protein-losing enteropathy, and protein-losing nephropathy.

Hyperproteinemia is seen with dehydration or chronic inflammatory disease (elevated globulins).

Glucose: 60–100 mg/dL normal range.

Hypoglycemia is seen with starvation, malnutrition, high-protein diets, severe hepatopathy, septicemia, and endocrinopathies.

Hyperglycemia may indicate diabetes mellitus.

Uric acid: 0–10 mg/dL normal range.

Hyperuricemia is seen with gout, severe renal disease, high-protein diets, or vitamin D_3 toxicity (from nephrocalcinosis).

AST (SGOT): <250 U/L is normal.

Elevated levels occur with tissue damage of skeletal or cardiac muscle or hepatic disease; toxemias and septicemias may cause elevated values due to generalized cell necrosis.

LDH: <1000 U/L is normal.

Elevated levels are seen in cases of generalized tissue damage (including RBC damage) due to its widespread distribution.

CPK: <1000 U/L is normal.

Elevated levels occur with skeletal muscle damage or injury.

Calcium: 8–20 mg/dL normal range.

Hypercalcemia is seen in ovulating females, and with increased dietary calcium and vitamin D_3, primary hyperparathyroidism, pseudohyperparathyroidism, and osteolytic bone lesions.

Hypocalcemia is seen with dietary imbalances of calcium, vitamin D_3, and phosphorus (metabolic bone disease may exhibit normocalcemia or hypocalcemia), and renal disease.

Phosphorus: 1–5 mg/dL normal range.

Hyperphosphatemia is seen in excess dietary phosphorus, renal disease, and hypervitaminosis D_3.

Hypophosphatemia is seen in anorexia, starvation, or nutritional imbalances.

Hepatic disease: Will usually see elevated AST and LDH but normal CPK.

Renal disease: May see increased uric acid but often will see increased phosphorus, decreased calcium, and a Ca:P ratio <1:1.

Note: The values given are ranges and will differ based upon the species involved as well as the laboratory used for blood analysis. As these values are ranges, they are meant to serve as a guideline to aid in interpreting serum chemistries in reptile patients.

Sources: Campbell, TW. Clinical pathology. In: Mader D. Reptile medicine and surgery. Philadelphia: WB Saunders, 1996:248–257; and Frye F. Reptile care: An atlas of diseases and treatments. Neptune City, NJ: TFH, 1991:209–280.

Index